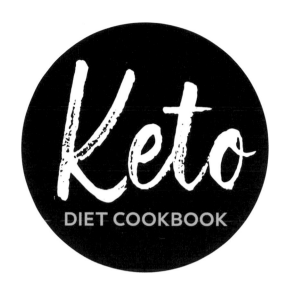

Keto

DIET COOKBOOK

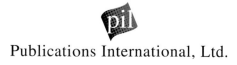

Publications International, Ltd.

Pictured on the front cover: Chicken Salad Bowl *(page 50)*.

Pictured on the back cover: Bacon Smashburger *(page 144)*.

Photograph on front cover and page 51 copyright © Shutterstock.com.

Contributing Writer: Jacqueline B. Marcus, MS, RDN, LDN, CNS, FADA, FAND

ISBN: 978-1-64030-830-5

Manufactured in China.

8 7 6 5 4 3 2 1

Let's get social!

 @Publications_International

 @PublicationsInternational

www.pilcookbooks.com

Contents

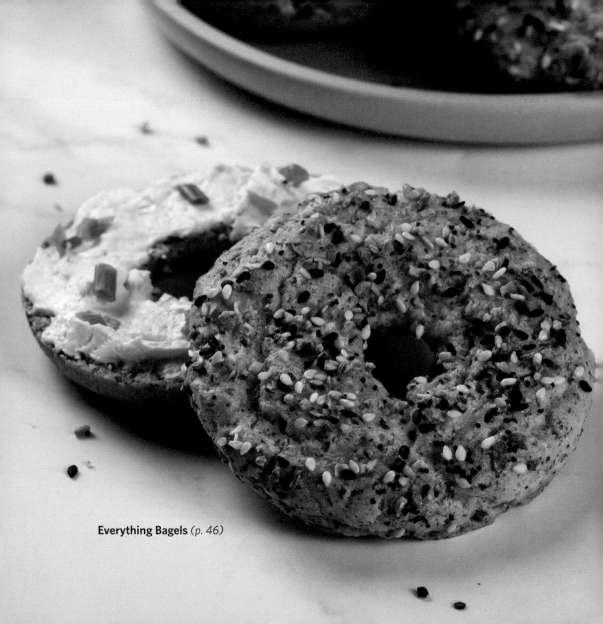

Everything Bagels *(p. 46)*

Introduction

Dietary Fats and Oils, Weight and Health

Want to hear some good news about dietary fats and oils—especially how they relate to weight and health?

Consuming dietary fats and oils is not as bad as you might think—nor will consuming dietary fats and oils necessarily make you fat. The right amounts and types of dietary fats and oils may actually be satisfying and contribute to weight loss and weight maintenance. Dietary fats and oils are essential to your overall diet. Understanding what dietary fats and oils are and how they fit into an overall diet will help you with food selection, preparation and meal and menu planning.

The keto diet is based on ketones, organic compounds that are produced when dietary carbohydrates are limited. Ketosis is a normal metabolic process whereby the body burns stored fats instead of glucose from carbohydrates for energy. A diet based on ketosis, with its abundance of dietary fats and oils may actually help your dieting efforts. Understanding more about ketones and their place in a ketogenic diet may assist your food choices and dietary efforts.

In addition to their role in weight loss and weight management, different types of dietary fats and oils and ketones are important for brain function, some disease protection and management, and overall health if used advantageously and correctly.

Dietary fats and oils are naturally found in foods and beverages such as dairy products, eggs, nuts, meats and seeds. Manufactured dietary fats and oils are found in some beverages, processed foods like margarine, cheeses and meats. Ketones are produced by the human body—you'll soon discover how.

There are differing viewpoints on the benefits of different types of dietary fats and oils and about ketones, the ideal amounts to consume and how ketones may sensibly be used for weight loss.

The purpose of this book is to help educate you about the types of dietary and blood fats and their contribution to health, and their relation to ketones and the ketogenic diet. It provides you with recipes that focus on healthy fats, proteins and non-starchy vegetables and de-emphasizes carbohydrates—particularly those that are refined or processed.

Your healthcare provider may help you determine if these approaches to eating and dieting are appropriate for you, so ask your doctor before you begin this or any other diet program.

CHOOSE THE RIGHT FATS

Fats are essential for proper body functioning and contribute satisfaction to diets, plus fats add flavor to foods and beverages. Still, fats provide more than twice the number of calories as carbohydrates or proteins (9 calories per gram compared to 4 calories per gram respectively). On a ketogenic diet, there is a different approach to fats than other diets that may restrict fats. The key is to understand the importance of fats in ketogenic diets and how to use them to your advantage.

TYPES OF FATS

Saturated fats are primarily found in foods from animal sources, such as meat, poultry and full-fat dairy products, while trans fats are mostly created when oils are partially hydrogenated to improve their cooking applications and to give them a longer shelf life. Saturated and trans fats may place a person at greater risk for heart disease. On the other hand, unsaturated fats that include monounsaturated and polyunsaturated fatty acids, found in plant-based foods such as avocados, nuts and seeds and olives and olive oil, and in fatty fish such as salmon, sardines and tuna tend to lower the risk of heart issues.

The American Heart Association (AHA) Diet and Lifestyle Recommendations suggest that a person limit saturated and trans fats and replace them with monounsaturated and polyunsaturated fats. If blood cholesterol needs to be lowered, then the recommendation is to reduce saturated fat to no more than 5 to 6 percent of total calories. For someone consuming 2,000 calories a day, this is about 13 grams of saturated fat, or about 117 calories. This is the equivalent of about 1 ounce of Cheddar cheese (9.4% total fat with 6 grams of saturated fat) and about 3 ounces of regular ground beef (25% total fat with 6.1 grams of saturated fat).

Try to eliminate trans fats (fats that have been processed into saturated fats) completely, or limit them to less than 1 percent of total daily calories. On a 2,000-calorie diet, this means that fewer than 20 calories (about 2 grams) should be derived from trans fats.

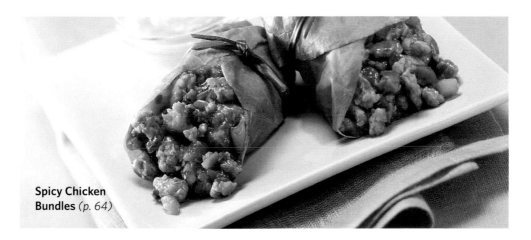

Spicy Chicken Bundles (p. 64)

The Ketogenic Diet and Dieting

The ketogenic diet is hardly new. The idea that fasting could be used as a therapy to treat disease was one that ancient Greek and Indian physicians embraced. "On the Sacred Disease," an early treatise in the Hippocratic Corpus, proposed how dietary modifications could be useful in epileptic management. Hippocrates, a Greek physician called the Father of Modern Medicine, wrote in "Epidemics" how abstinence from food and drink cured epilepsy.

In the 20th century, the first ketogenic diet became popularized in the 1920's and 30's as a regimen for treating epilepsy and an alternative to non-mainstream fasting. It was also promoted as a means of restoring health. In 1921, the ketogenic diet was officially established when an endocrinologist noted that three water-soluble compounds were produced by the liver as a result of following a diet that was rich in fat and low in carbohydrates. The term "water diet" had been used prior to this time to describe a diet that was free of starch and sugar. This is because when carbohydrates are broken down by the body carbon dioxide and water are by-products. When newer, anticonvulsant therapies were established, the ketogenic diet was temporarily abandoned.

In the 1960's the ketogenic diet was revisited when it was noted that more ketones are produced by medium chain triglycerides (MCTs) per unit of energy than by normal dietary fats (mostly long-chain triglycerides) because MCTs are quickly transported to the liver to be metabolized. In research diets where about 60 percent of the calories came from MCT oil, more protein and up to about three times as many carbohydrates could be consumed in comparison to "classic" ketogenic diets. This is why MCT oil is included in some ketogenic diets today.

In the 1950's and 1960's many versions of the ketogenic diet were popularized as high-protein, low-carbohydrate and a quick method of weight loss. Also at this time, the risk factors of excess fat and protein in the diet were criticized for being detrimental to health.

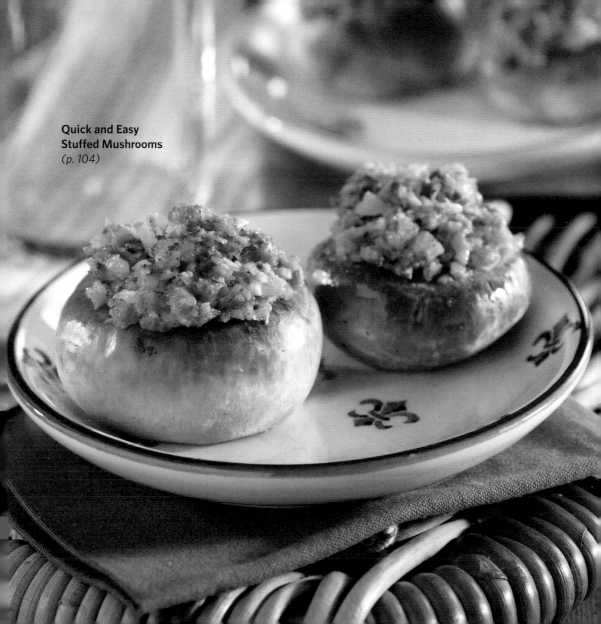

**Quick and Easy
Stuffed Mushrooms**
(p. 104)

Outside of the medical community, the ketogenic diet was not widely recognized for its therapeutic benefits so response to it was sensational in scope.

Then in the 1980's the Glycemic Index (GI) of foods and beverages was revealed that accounted for the differences in the speed of digestion of different types of carbohydrates. This explanation became the springboard for a number of ketogenic diets that were revised from years earlier. By the late 1990's the low-carb craze became one of the most popular types of dieting. Since this time, the original ketogenic diet underwent many refinements and hybrid diets developed.

Variations of the ketogenic diet continued to surface throughout the 20th century since the premise of the ketogenic diet—higher fat and protein and low carbohydrate—was used to treat diabetes and induce weight loss among other applications.

Table 1 summarizes the ketogenic diet basics. Many clinical studies examined their effectiveness and safety and their advantages and drawbacks were identified. These are condensed in **Table 2.**

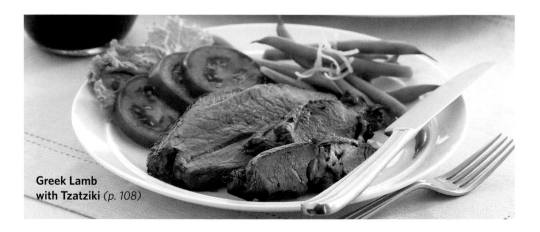

Greek Lamb with Tzatziki (p. 108)

TABLE 1

KETOGENIC DIET BASICS

Generally, the percentages of macronutrients on a ketogenic diet are as follows:

- **Fat** 60 to 75 percent of total daily calories
- **Protein** 15 to 30 percent of total daily calories
- **Carbohydrates** 5 to 10 percent of total daily calories

Both fat and protein have high priority on a ketogenic diet, with non-starchy carbohydrates completing the remaining calories. While calories are not as important on the ketogenic diet as they are for other diets, a closer examination of the contributions of these macronutrients helps to put the amounts into perspective.

If total daily calories were about 2,000, then the percentages of macronutrients on a ketogenic diet would resemble the following amounts:

- **Fat** 60 to 75 percent of total daily calories or about 1,200 to 1,500 calories
- **Protein** 15 to 30 percent of total daily calories or about 300 to 600 calories
- **Carbohydrates** 5 to 10 percent of total daily calories or about 100 to 200 calories

In selecting foods and beverages, think protein and fat first, then non-starchy carbohydrates to complete. Until you truly have a handle on what constitutes low carbohydrates, find a carbohydrate counter to help to keep you in line. The ketogenic diet meal suggestions in **Table 5 – SAMPLE KETOGENIC DIET MEALS: BREAKFAST, LUNCH, DINNER AND SNACKS** on pages 28 and 29 may help your food and beverage selections.

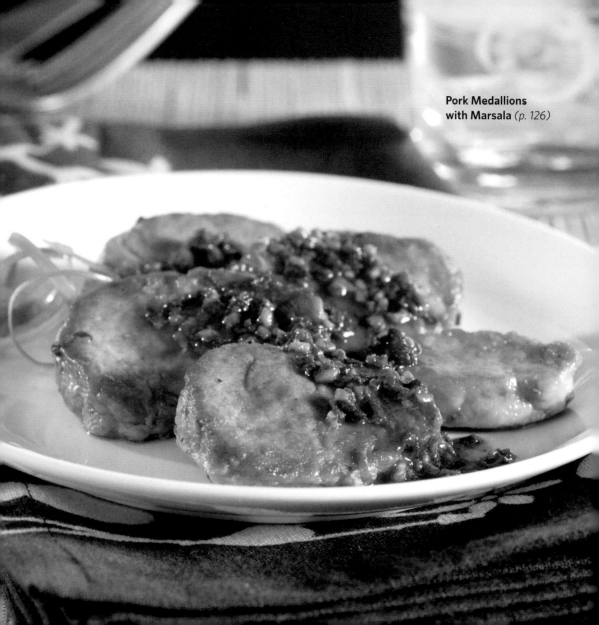

**Pork Medallions
with Marsala** *(p. 126)*

TABLE 2

ADVANTAGES AND DRAWBACKS OF KETOGENIC DIETS

ADVANTAGES

- No calorie counting or focus on portion sizes
- Initial weight loss
- After initial transition, hunger subsides
- Improved energy
- Improved blood pressure
- Improved blood fats: high-density lipoproteins, cholesterol, low-density lipoproteins, triglycerides
- Reduced blood sugar, C-reactive protein (marker of inflammation), insulin, waist circumference
- Significant short-term weight loss possible

DRAWBACKS

- Hard to sustain
- Limited food choices
- May lead to taste fatigue
- Socialization difficult
- Digestive issues (such as constipation, fatty stool, nausea)
- Nutrient deficiencies (such as calcium, vitamins A, C and D, B-vitamins, fiber, magnesium, selenium)
- Fiber, vitamin and mineral supplements suggested
- Increased urination (bladder, kidney contraindications)
- Diabetes issues
- Rapid, sizeable short-term weight loss concerning; long-term weight maintenance questionable

Fat in Health and Disease

Fats are essential to the diet and health for many purposes. Fats function as the body's thermostat. The layer of fat just beneath the skin helps to keep the body warm or causes it to perspire to cool the body.

Fat contributes to bile acids, cell membranes and steroid hormones (such as estrogen and testosterone), cushions the body from shock and helps to regulate fluid balance. Too many or too few fats in the diet may influence each of these important body functions.

One of the most important roles of fat in the body is as an energy source, especially when carbohydrates are not available from the diet or are lacking in the body. When people did manual work all day and expended the calories that they consumed, they made good use of carbohydrates and fats in their diet and within their energy stores. Today's laborsaving devices and sedentary lifestyles create less need for excess carbohydrate calories— particularly if they are refined. Even a plant-based diet may be unnecessarily high in refined carbohydrate calories.

Over the years, as humans moved from a plant-based diet toward an animal-based diet, the composition of fatty acids in the American diet switched from monounsaturated and polyunsaturated fats to more saturated fats, which are associated more with cardiovascular disease. A diet that is only filled with saturated fats may not be healthy. Incorporating avocado, fish, nuts, oils and seeds and other foods that contain monounsaturated and polyunsaturated fats into your diet may help to support a healthier proportion of fats in the body for weight maintenance and good health.

Besides cardiovascular disease, excess saturated and trans fats in the human diet are associated with certain cancers, cerebral vascular disease, diabetes, obesity and metabolic syndrome (a collection of conditions that may include abnormal cholesterol or triglyceride levels, excess body fat around the waist, high blood sugar and increased blood pressure that may increase a person's risk of diabetes, heart disease and/or stroke).

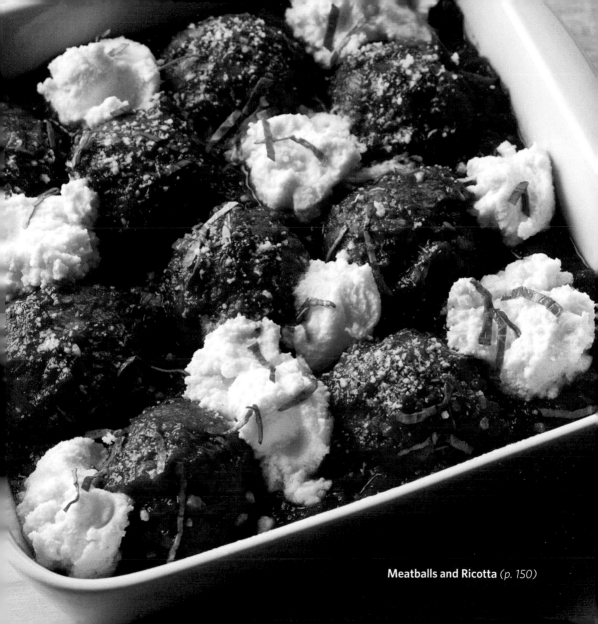

Meatballs and Ricotta *(p. 150)*

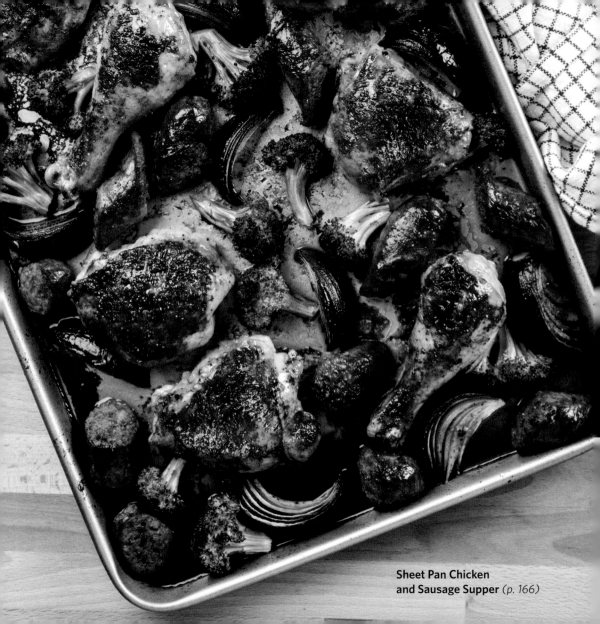

Sheet Pan Chicken and Sausage Supper (*p. 166*)

THE CHOLESTEROL CONTROVERSY

Atherosclerosis, or hardening of the arteries, is not a modern disease. Rather, the association between blood cholesterol and cardiovascular disease was recognized as far back as the 1850's.

One hundred years later in the 1950's, cholesterol and saturated fats in the diet were implicated as major risk factors for cardiovascular disease. Then in the 1980's, major US health institutions established that the process of lowering blood cholesterol (specifically LDL-cholesterol) reduces the risk of heart attacks that are caused by coronary heart disease.

Some scientists questioned this conclusion that marked the unofficial start of what's been called the "cholesterol controversy." Studies of cholesterol-lowering drugs known as statins supported the idea that reducing blood cholesterol means less mortality from heart disease. Subsequent statin studies have questioned this association. Other factors aside from dietary cholesterol have since been identified that may lead to elevated blood cholesterol, such as trans fats.

The liver manufactures cholesterol, so reducing cholesterol in the diet should help to reduce blood cholesterol, coronary heart disease and the risk of heart attack. But in some individuals, the liver produces more cholesterol than the body requires and cardiovascular disease may still develop. Accordingly, dietary cholesterol does not necessarily predict cardiovascular disease or a heart attack.

While dietary cholesterol may be a measure for greater cardiovascular risks, cardiovascular disease and heart attacks are also dependent upon such lifestyle and genetic factors as age, diet, exercise, gender, genetics, medication and stress. Reducing hydrogenated fats, saturated fats and trans fats; incorporating mono- and polyunsaturated fats and losing weight to help better manage blood fats are other sensible measures to take.

Longer-term weight management is also a preventative measure in cardiovascular disease. Reducing cholesterol and saturated fat in the diet while integrating foods and beverages with mono- and polyunsaturated fats and oils, dietary fiber, antioxidants and other phytonutrients may lead to a decrease in overall calorie consumption and weight loss and an improvement in overall health.

So What (and How) Should I Eat?

If you want to lose body fat, then the general consensus is that you need to take in fewer calories than you burn for energy. For example, if you're an average woman over 40, decreasing your caloric intake may be a reasonable starting point. If you are of shorter stature and/or very inactive, or you haven't dropped any pounds after a few weeks, you may consider lowering your daily intake of calories by 100-calorie increments until you start seeing weight loss. But don't go much below 1,000 calories without your health care provider's supervision. (And be sure to check with your health care provider before making any major changes to your diet or activity level, especially if you have any serious health problems.)

Another approach to weight loss is the ketogenic diet that does not focus on calories. Instead, the ketogenic diet focuses on the composition of calories from fats, proteins and carbohydrates.

> **THE KEY IS TO UNDERSTAND THE IMPORTANCE OF FATS IN KETOGENIC DIETS AND HOW TO USE THEM TO YOUR ADVANTAGE.**

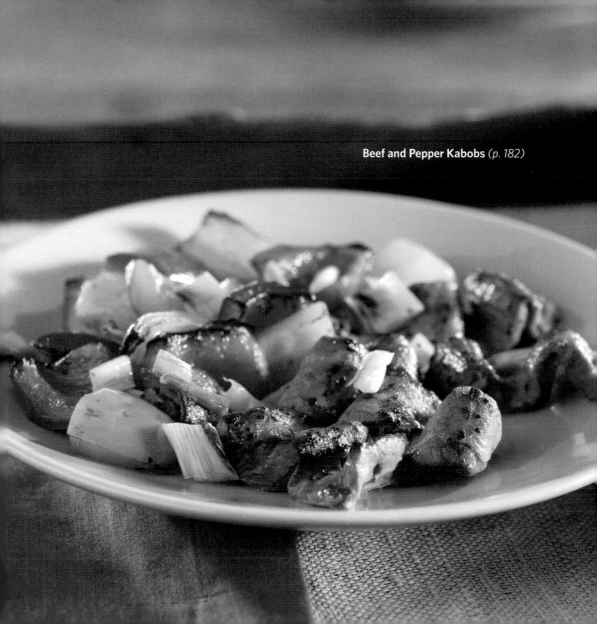

Beef and Pepper Kabobs *(p. 182)*

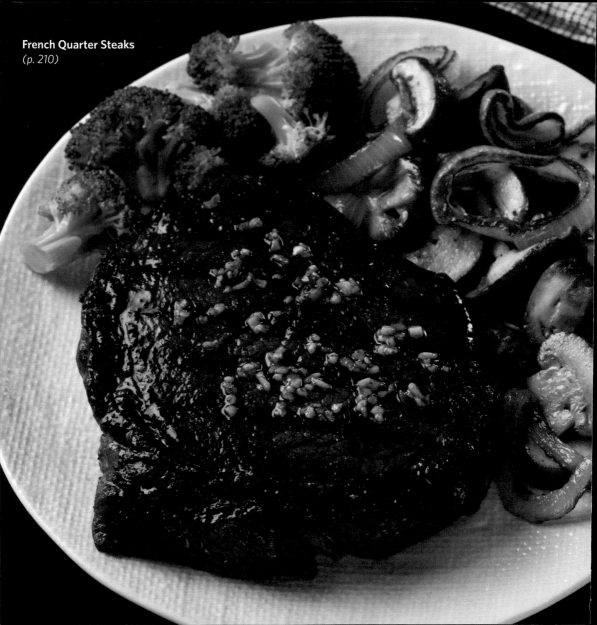

French Quarter Steaks
(p. 210)

Fats are satisfying because they take longer for the body to digest, and some are converted into ketones for energy. You don't want to skimp on proteins because protein helps maintain and build calorie-burning muscle and also keeps you satiated between meals. Choose protein sources that supply monounsaturated fats and other heart-healthy unsaturated fats; good options include fish, seafood, nuts and seeds. (Fatty fish, such as herring, mackerel, salmon and tuna contain polyunsaturated fats—especially disease-fighting omega-3 fatty acids). You'll need to replace highly processed and refined foods that are full of saturated and trans fats, sugar and refined carbohydrates with minimally processed fiber- and nutrient-rich foods that include non-starchy vegetables.

What you'll likely end up with is a satisfying eating plan with ample protein, healthy fats and minimal carbohydrates that may help you to feel full and lose weight in the process. It's also a plan that may help you to maintain weight loss over time in a modified manner.

If you've ever tried to lose weight before, you know how quickly between-meal hunger may sabotage your best efforts. When your stomach starts rumbling hours before your next meal, it's tempting to grab whatever is available. Often, that "whatever" is some unhealthy packaged snack food or beverage that is loaded with empty calories, sodium, sugars and/or unhealthy fats. Or, if you manage to ignore this hunger, you may become so ravenous at the next meal that you consume far more calories than your body actually needs.

WHAT YOU'LL LIKELY END UP WITH IS A SATISFYING EATING PLAN WITH AMPLE PROTEIN, HEALTHY FATS AND MINIMAL CARBOHYDRATES THAT MAY HELP YOU TO FEEL FULL AND LOSE WEIGHT IN THE PROCESS.

To prevent hunger from spoiling your weight-loss efforts, eat when you are hungry and stop eating when you are full, whether a meal or snack. Try to consume meals and snacks that include a source of hunger-fighting protein and healthy fat, and count your carbs so as not to exceed the daily limit of 20 to 50 grams of non-starchy carbohydrates.

Drink plenty of water throughout the day (especially if you live in a hot climate or sweat excessively) since ketogenic diets tend to be dehydrating and may lead to fatigue or ill feelings. This may be due to an imbalance of electrolytes; specifically sodium that the kidneys excrete during ketosis. Sometimes lightly salting your food may help to restore sodium. A high-quality vitamin and mineral supplement is also sensible.

Notes on Ketogenic Foods, Beverages and Ingredients

In general, the foods, beverages and ingredients that are included in a ketogenic diet incorporate eggs, healthy fats and oils, fish, meats and organ meats and non-starchy vegetables. These "acceptable" foods, beverages and ingredients contain protein and fats and are low in carbohydrates that contribute to the effectiveness of ketogenic diets. They are listed in **Table 3 – ACCEPTABLE FOODS, BEVERAGES AND INGREDIENTS FOR KETOGENIC DIETS.**

In **Table 4 – UNACCEPTABLE FOODS, BEVERAGES AND INGREDIENTS FOR KETOGENIC DIETS** are shown. While there is a wide-range of ketogenic diet approaches, these foods, beverages and ingredients are generally considered to be "unacceptable" on many ketogenic diets. In general, their carbohydrate content exceeds what is considered as optimal for effective ketosis and diet success.

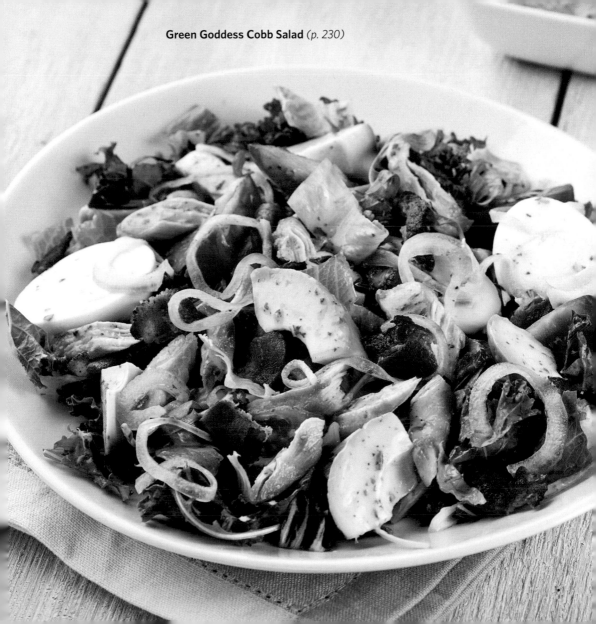

Green Goddess Cobb Salad *(p. 230)*

TABLE 3

ACCEPTABLE FOODS, BEVERAGES AND INGREDIENTS FOR KETOGENIC DIETS

BEVERAGES
- Broth
- Hard liquor
- Nut milks
- Unsweetened coffee, tea
- Water

EGGS
- Egg whites
- Powdered eggs
- Whole eggs

FATS AND OILS
- Butter
- Cocoa butter
- Coconut butter, cream and oil
- Ghee
- Lard
- Oils: avocado oil, macadamia nut oil, MCT oil, olive oil and cold-pressed vegetable oils (flax, safflower, soybean)
- Mayonnaise

DAIRY PRODUCTS
- Crème fraîche
- Greek yogurt
- Hard cheese (aged Cheddar, feta, Parmesan, Swiss)
- Heavy cream
- Soft cheese (Brie, blue, Colby, Monterey Jack, mozzarella)
- Sour cream
- Spreadable cheese (cream cheese, cottage cheese and mascarpone)

FISH AND SEAFOOD
- Anchovies
- Fish (catfish, cod, flounder, halibut, mackerel, mahi-mahi, salmon, snapper, trout, tuna)
- Shellfish (clams, crab, lobster, mussels, oysters, scallops, squid)

MEATS AND POULTRY
- Beef (ground beef, roasts, steak, stew meat)
- Goat
- Lamb (leg, loin, rack, ribs, shank, shoulder)
- Organ meats (heart, kidneys, liver, tongue)
- Poultry with skin (such as chicken, duck, pheasant, quail, turkey)
- Pork (bacon and sausage without fillers, ground pork, ham, pork chops, pork loin, tenderloin)
- Tofu used in moderation in some keto diets)

TABLE 3 (CONTINUED)

- Veal (double, flank, leg, rib, shoulder, sirloin)

NON-DAIRY BEVERAGES

- Almond milk
- Cashew milk
- Coconut milk
- Soymilk (used in moderation in some keto diets)

NUTS AND SEEDS

- Nut butters (almond, macadamia)
- Seeds (chia, flax, poppy, sesame, sunflower)
- Whole nuts (almonds, Brazil nuts, macadamia, pecans, hazelnuts, pine nuts, walnuts)

PANTRY ITEMS

- Herbs (dried or fresh such as basil, cilantro, oregano, parsley, rosemary and thyme)
- Horseradish
- Hot sauce
- Ketchup (unsweetened)
- Mustard
- Pepper
- Pesto sauce
- Pickles
- Salad dressings (without sweeteners)
- Salt
- Spices (such as ground red pepper, chili powder, cinnamon and cumin)

- Unsweetened gelatin
- Vinegar
- Whey protein (unsweetened)
- Worcestershire sauce

VEGETABLES

- Avocados
- Cruciferous vegetables (broccoli, brussels sprouts, cabbage, cauliflower, kohlrabi)
- Fermented vegetables (kimchi, sauerkraut)
- Leafy greens (bok choy, chard, endive, lettuce, kale, radicchio, spinach, watercress)

- Lemon and lime juice and peel
- Mushrooms
- Non-starchy vegetables (asparagus, bamboo shoots, celery, cucumber)
- Seaweed and kelp
- Squash (spaghetti squash, yellow squash, zucchini)
- Tomatoes (used in moderation in some keto diets)

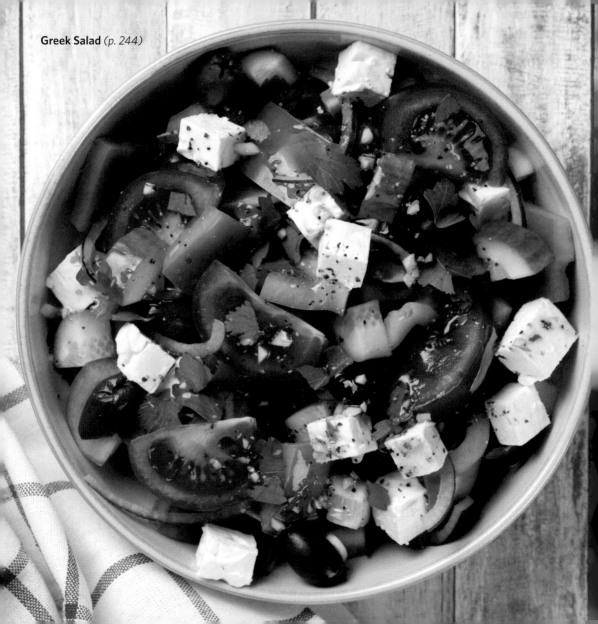

Greek Salad *(p. 244)*

TABLE 4

UNACCEPTABLE FOODS, BEVERAGES AND INGREDIENTS FOR KETOGENIC DIETS

- Alcohol other than hard liquor (beer, sugary alcoholic beverages, wine)
- Beans
- Breads and breadstuffs
- Cakes and pastries
- Candy
- Cereals
- Cookies
- Crackers
- Flours
- Fruit, all (fresh, dried)
- Grains (amaranth, barley, buckwheat, bulgur, corn, millet, oats, rice, rye, sorghum, sprouted grains, wheat)
- Legumes (lentils, peas)
- Margarines with trans fats
- Milk (full-fat milk is acceptable in some ketogenic diets)
- Oats and muesli
- Potatoes, all kinds (white, yellow, sweet)
- Quinoa
- Pasta
- Pizza
- Processed and refined snack foods
- Rice
- Root vegetables
- Soda
- Sports drinks
- Sugar and honey
- Syrup
- Wheat gluten
- Yams

TABLE 5

SAMPLE KETOGENIC DIET MEALS: BREAKFAST, LUNCH, DINNER AND SNACKS

Examples of combinations of protein, low-carb, non-starchy vegetables and fats:

BREAKFAST:

- Almond, coconut, hemp or other nut or seed milks or beverages (unsweetened)

- Bacon, sausage or sliced meats (without carbohydrate fillers)

- Cheese, hard or soft varieties

- Eggs, scrambled or fried + vegetables (asparagus, broccoli, garlic, mushrooms, onions or spinach) + coconut or olive oil + avocado, olives, salsa and/or sour cream

- Greek yogurt with nut butter, chia or flax seeds, herbs and spices (cinnamon, ginger or nutmeg)

- Smoked fish (such as lox, sable or whitefish)

- Smoothies made with keto-friendly ingredients (protein powder, almond or coconut butter, avocado, cocoa powder, chia or flax seeds, spices such as cinnamon, smoked paprika or turmeric and unsweetened almond or hemp milk)

- Vegetable slices (cucumber or zucchini or lettuce) topped with cheese

LUNCH AND DINNER:

- Eggs + watercress or spinach + avocado dressing

- Lamb + kale + sesame oil

- Pork + cauliflower + coconut butter

- Poultry + zucchini and yellow squash + extra virgin olive oil

TABLE 5 *(CONTINUED)*

- Salmon + broccoli + mustard sauce
- Sardines + cucumbers and onions + sour cream dressing
- Seafood + leafy green salad + oil and vinegar dressing
- Steak + asparagus + butter sauce
- Tofu + mushrooms and bok choy + ghee
- Tuna + celery + mayonnaise

SNACKS:

- Asparagus with goat cheese dip
- Avocado filled hard-cooked eggs
- Celery + nut or seed butter
- Cheese + olive skewers
- Chia and flaxseed crackers + cream cheese
- Cucumber and cream cheese spread
- Cream cheese and bacon stuffed celery
- Deviled eggs with fresh herbs and chives
- Greek yogurt with chopped cucumbers and garlic
- Guacamole with onions and garlic
- Ham and Cheddar or Swiss cheese roll ups
- Mixed nut-coated cheese balls
- Nut butters (such as almond) blended with ricotta cheese
- Olives stuffed with blue cheese
- Parmesan cheese crisps
- Seeds and seed butters such as tahini
- Sliced jicama with herbed cream cheese

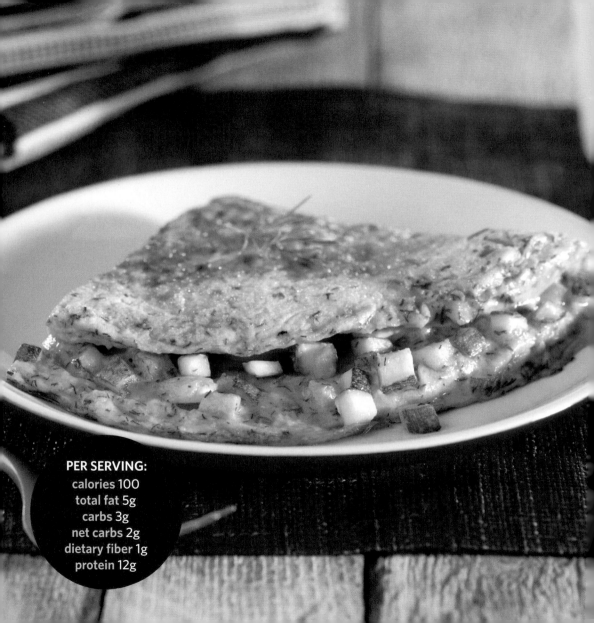

PER SERVING:
calories 100
total fat 5g
carbs 3g
net carbs 2g
dietary fiber 1g
protein 12g

Breakfast

Zucchini-Dill Omelet

MAKES 2 SERVINGS

1 egg*

4 egg whites*

2 tablespoons milk

½ teaspoon dried dill weed

¼ teaspoon salt

⅛ teaspoon black pepper

1 teaspoon butter

1 cup diced zucchini

Or use 4 whole eggs instead of 1 whole egg and 4 egg whites.

1. Whisk egg, egg whites, milk, dill, salt and pepper in medium bowl until blended.

2. Spray medium nonstick skillet with nonstick cooking spray. Add butter; melt over medium-high heat. Add zucchini; cook 4 minutes or until lightly browned, stirring occasionally. Add egg mixture; cook until edges are set. Push edges toward center with spatula and tilt pan allowing uncooked portion to flow underneath. When eggs are set, fold omelet over and cut in half.

Feta Brunch Bake

MAKES 4 SERVINGS

6 eggs

2 packages (10 ounces each) frozen chopped spinach, thawed and squeezed dry

1½ cups (6 ounces) crumbled feta cheese

⅓ cup chopped onion

1 jarred roasted red pepper, chopped

2 tablespoons chopped fresh parsley

¼ teaspoon salt

¼ teaspoon dried dill weed

Dash black pepper

1. Preheat oven to 400°F. Spray 1-quart baking dish with nonstick cooking spray.

2. Whisk eggs in large bowl until foamy. Stir in spinach, cheese, onion, roasted pepper, parsley, salt, dill and black pepper. Pour into prepared baking dish.

3. Bake 20 minutes or until set. Let stand 5 minutes before serving. Cut evenly into 4 squares to serve.

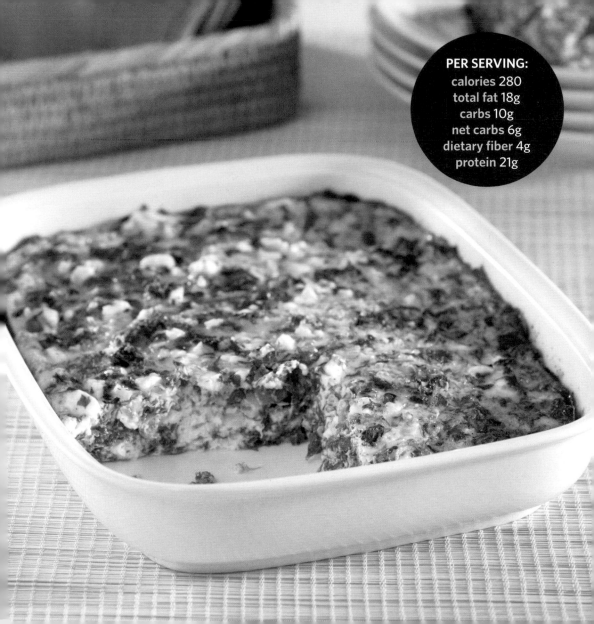

PER SERVING:
calories 280
total fat 18g
carbs 10g
net carbs 6g
dietary fiber 4g
protein 21g

Spinach, Pepper and Olive Omelet

MAKES 4 SERVINGS

1 cup diced red bell pepper

½ teaspoon dried rosemary

⅛ teaspoon red pepper flakes

2 cups loosely packed baby spinach (2 ounces total), coarsely chopped

16 stuffed green olives, such as manzanilla, sliced

2 tablespoons chopped fresh basil

2 cups liquid egg substitute *or* 8 whole eggs, beaten

3 tablespoons milk

2 ounces crumbled goat cheese or feta cheese, divided

1. Spray medium nonstick skillet with nonstick cooking spray; heat over medium-high heat. Add bell pepper, rosemary and red pepper flakes; cook and stir 4 minutes or until soft. Remove from heat. Stir in spinach, olives and basil; toss gently. Place in medium bowl; cover to allow spinach to wilt slightly.

2. Combine egg substitute and milk in another medium bowl; whisk until well blended. Wipe out skillet with paper towel. Spray skillet with cooking spray; heat over medium heat. Pour half of egg mixture into skillet. Cook 3 to 5 minutes, gently lifting edge of eggs with spatula to allow uncooked portion to flow underneath.

3. When egg mixture is set, spoon half of spinach mixture over half of omelet. Top with half of cheese. Loosen omelet with spatula and fold in half. Slide omelet onto serving plate and cover with foil to keep warm. Repeat with remaining ingredients. Cut omelets in half to serve.

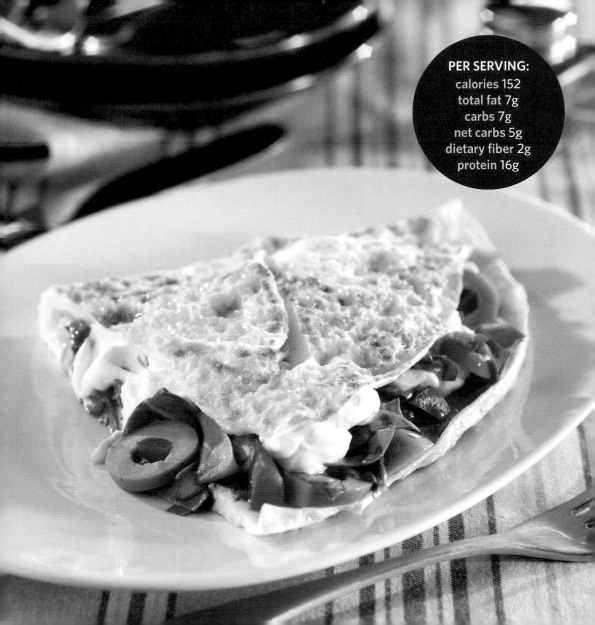

PER SERVING:
calories 152
total fat 7g
carbs 7g
net carbs 5g
dietary fiber 2g
protein 16g

Joe's Special

MAKES 4 SERVINGS

1 pound lean ground beef
2 cups sliced mushrooms
1 small onion, chopped
2 teaspoons Worcestershire sauce
1 teaspoon dried oregano
1 teaspoon ground nutmeg
½ teaspoon garlic powder
½ teaspoon salt
1 package (10 ounces) frozen chopped spinach, thawed
4 eggs, lightly beaten
⅓ cup grated Parmesan cheese

1. Spray large skillet with nonstick cooking spray; heat over medium-high heat. Add ground beef, mushrooms and onion; cook and stir 6 to 8 minutes or until meat is browned. Add Worcestershire sauce, oregano, nutmeg, garlic powder and salt.

2. Drain spinach (do not squeeze dry); stir into meat mixture. Push mixture to one side of pan. Reduce heat to medium. Pour eggs into other side of pan; cook without stirring 1 to 2 minutes or until set on bottom. Lift eggs with spatula to allow uncooked portion to flow underneath. Repeat until softly set. Gently stir into meat mixture and heat through. Stir in cheese.

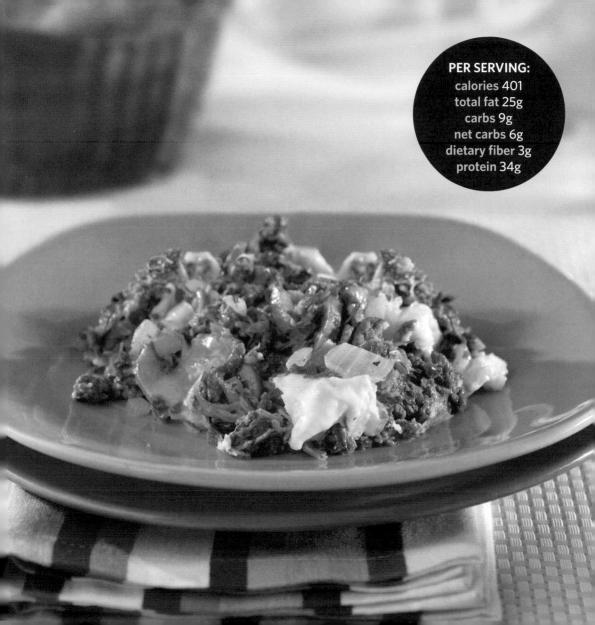

PER SERVING:
calories 401
total fat 25g
carbs 9g
net carbs 6g
dietary fiber 3g
protein 34g

Smoked Salmon and Spinach Frittata

MAKES 6 TO 8 SERVINGS

2 tablespoons vegetable or olive oil, divided
1 medium red onion, diced
1 clove garlic, minced
1 package (5 ounces) fresh baby spinach
10 eggs

1 teaspoon dried dill weed
¼ teaspoon salt
¼ teaspoon black pepper
4 ounces smoked salmon, chopped
4 ounces aged Cheddar cheese, cut into ¼-inch cubes

1. Position oven rack in upper-middle position. Preheat broiler.

2. Heat 1 tablespoon oil in large ovenproof nonstick skillet. Add onion; cook 7 to 8 minutes or until softened, stirring occasionally. Add garlic; cook and stir 1 minute. Add spinach; cook 3 minutes or just until wilted. Transfer mixture to small bowl.

3. Whisk eggs, dill, salt and pepper in large bowl until blended. Stir in salmon, cheese and spinach mixture.

4. Heat remaining 1 tablespoon oil in same skillet over medium heat. Add egg mixture; cook about 3 minutes, stirring gently to form large curds. Cook without stirring 5 minutes or until eggs are just beginning to set.

5. Transfer skillet to oven. Broil 2 to 3 minutes or until frittata is puffed, set and lightly browned. Let stand 5 minutes; carefully slide frittata onto large plate or cutting board. Cut into wedges.

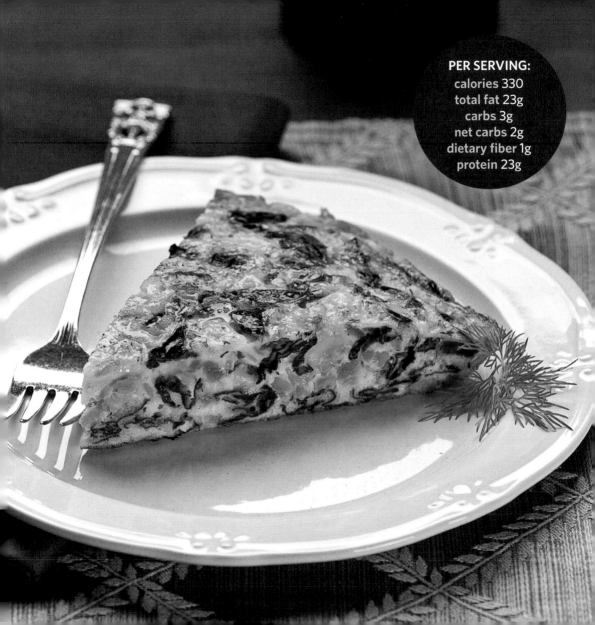

Ham and Vegetable Omelet

MAKES 4 SERVINGS

2 ounces diced ham (about ½ cup)

1 small onion, diced

½ medium green bell pepper, diced

½ medium red bell pepper, diced

2 cloves garlic, minced

1½ cups liquid egg substitute *or* 6 eggs, beaten

⅛ teaspoon black pepper

½ cup (2 ounces) shredded Colby cheese, divided

1 medium tomato, chopped

Hot pepper sauce (optional)

1. Spray 12-inch nonstick skillet with nonstick cooking spray; heat over medium-high heat. Add ham, onion, bell peppers and garlic; cook and stir 5 minutes or until vegetables are crisp-tender. Transfer mixture to large bowl.

2. Wipe out skillet with paper towels; spray with cooking spray. Heat over medium-high heat. Pour egg substitute into skillet; sprinkle with black pepper. Cook 2 minutes or until bottom is set, lifting edge of egg with spatula to allow uncooked portion to flow underneath. Reduce heat to medium-low; cover and cook 4 minutes or until top is set.

3. Gently slide omelet onto large serving plate; spoon ham mixture down center. Sprinkle with ¼ cup cheese. Carefully fold two sides of omelet over ham mixture; sprinkle with remaining ¼ cup cheese and tomato. Cut into 4 pieces; serve immediately with hot pepper sauce, if desired.

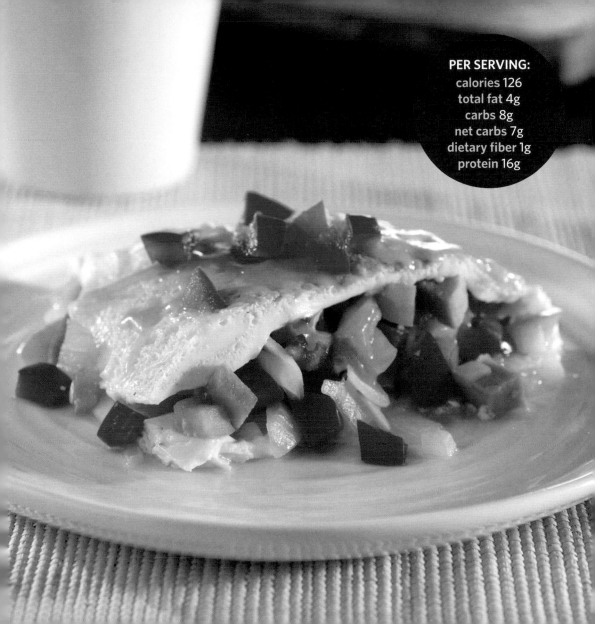

PER SERVING:
calories 126
total fat 4g
carbs 8g
net carbs 7g
dietary fiber 1g
protein 16g

Spicy Scrambled Eggs with Tomatoes

MAKES 4 SERVINGS

8 eggs
½ teaspoon salt
2 tablespoons butter
2 tablespoons vegetable oil
⅓ cup finely chopped onion

2 to 4 fresh serrano peppers, finely chopped
2 medium tomatoes, seeded, chopped and drained

1. Whisk eggs and salt in medium bowl.

2. Heat butter and oil in large skillet over medium heat. Add onion and peppers; cook and stir 45 seconds or until hot but not soft. Stir in tomatoes. Increase heat to medium-high; cook and stir 45 seconds or until tomatoes are hot.

3. Add egg mixture to skillet. Cook without stirring 1 minute. Cook 2 to 3 minutes more, stirring lightly until eggs are softly set.

NOTE: For milder flavor, remove the seeds from some or all of the peppers.

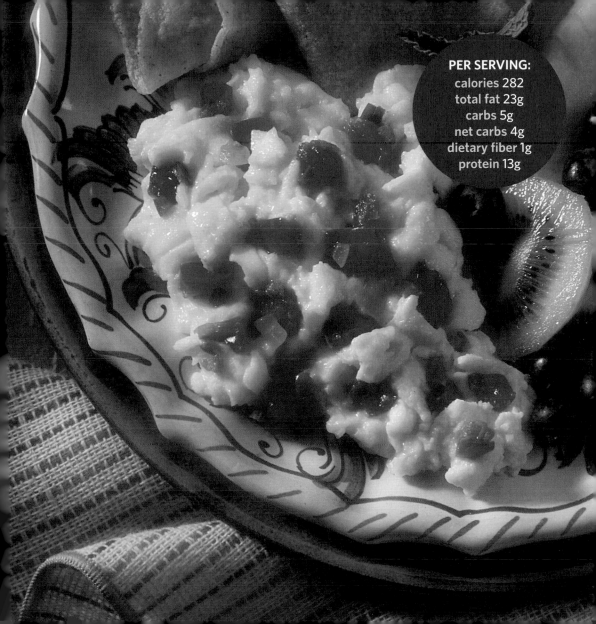

PER SERVING:
calories 282
total fat 23g
carbs 5g
net carbs 4g
dietary fiber 1g
protein 13g

Sausage and Cheddar Omelet

MAKES 4 SERVINGS

2 uncooked turkey breakfast sausage links (about 1 ounce each)

1 small onion, diced

1½ cups liquid egg substitute *or* 6 eggs, lightly beaten

⅛ teaspoon salt

¼ teaspoon black pepper

½ cup (2 ounces) shredded Cheddar cheese, divided

Sliced green onions (optional)

1. Heat 12-inch nonstick skillet over medium-high heat. Remove sausage from casings. Add sausage and diced onion to skillet. Cook about 5 minutes or until sausage is no longer pink and onion is crisp-tender, stirring to break up meat. Transfer to plate.

2. Wipe out skillet with paper towels; spray with nonstick cooking spray. Heat over medium-high heat. Pour egg substitute into skillet; sprinkle with salt and pepper. Cook 2 minutes or until bottom is set, lifting edge of egg with spatula to allow uncooked portion to flow underneath. Reduce heat to medium-low. Cover; cook 4 minutes or until top is set.

3. Gently slide cooked egg onto large serving plate; spoon sausage mixture down center. Sprinkle with ¼ cup cheese. Fold sides of omelet over sausage mixture. Sprinkle with remaining ¼ cup cheese and garnish with green onions. Cut into 4 pieces; serve immediately.

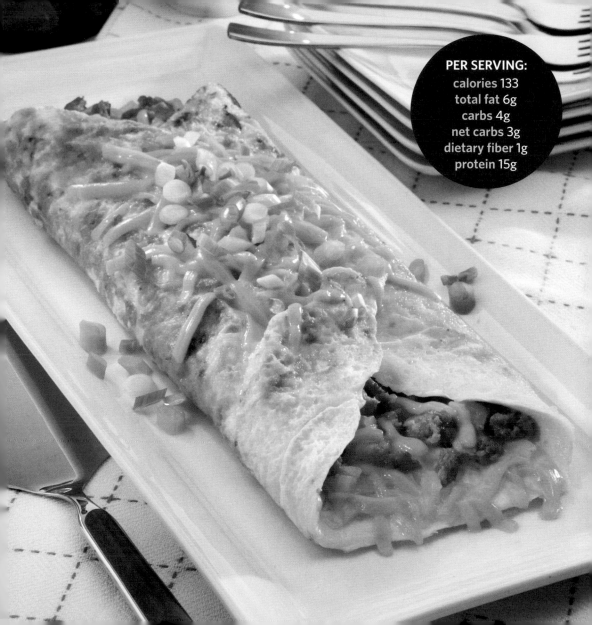

PER SERVING:
calories 133
total fat 6g
carbs 4g
net carbs 3g
dietary fiber 1g
protein 15g

Everything Bagels

MAKES 12 BAGELS

6 eggs, at room temperature, separated
¼ teaspoon cream of tartar
2 cups almond flour
3½ teaspoons baking powder
½ teaspoon salt
¼ teaspoon garlic powder
6 tablespoons butter, melted and cooled slightly
½ cup finely shredded Asiago cheese
2 tablespoons everything bagel seasoning

1. Preheat oven to 350°F. Spray 12 cavities of doughnut pans with nonstick cooking spray.

2. Place egg whites and cream of tartar in large bowl; attach whisk attachment to stand mixer. Whip egg whites on high speed 2 minutes or until stiff peaks form. Transfer egg whites to medium bowl.

3. Combine almond flour, baking powder, salt and garlic powder in mixer bowl. Add melted butter and egg yolks; mix on medium speed until well blended. Add cheese; mix well.

4. Stir one third of egg whites into almond flour mixture with spatula until well blended. Gently fold in remaining egg whites until thoroughly blended. Scoop mixture into large resealable food storage bag; cut off one corner. Pipe about ¼ cup batter into each doughnut cavity. Sprinkle each with ½ teaspoon everything bagel seasoning.

5. Bake about 10 minutes or until bagels are golden brown and set. Cool in pans 2 minutes. Remove to wire rack; serve warm or cool completely.

EVERYTHING BAGEL MUFFINS: If you don't have doughnut pans or would prefer to make muffins instead, scoop batter into 12 greased standard muffin pan cups. Sprinkle with bagel seasoning. Bake 15 minutes or until tops are golden brown and toothpick inserted into centers comes out clean.

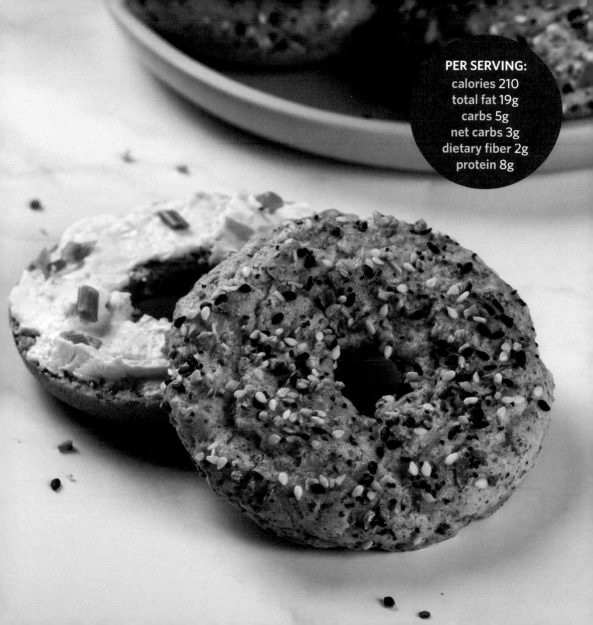

PER SERVING:
calories 210
total fat 19g
carbs 5g
net carbs 3g
dietary fiber 2g
protein 8g

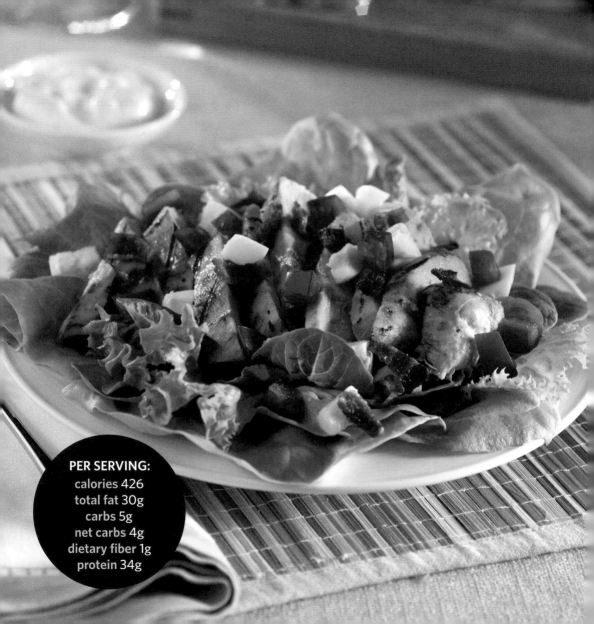

PER SERVING:
calories 426
total fat 30g
carbs 5g
net carbs 4g
dietary fiber 1g
protein 34g

Lunch

BLT Chicken Salad for Two

MAKES 2 SERVINGS

2 boneless skinless chicken breasts
¼ cup mayonnaise
½ teaspoon black pepper
4 large lettuce leaves
1 large tomato, seeded and diced

3 slices bacon, crisp-cooked and crumbled
1 hard-cooked egg, chopped
   Additional mayonnaise or ranch dressing (optional)

1. Prepare grill for direct cooking.

2. Brush chicken with ¼ cup mayonnaise; sprinkle with pepper. Grill over medium heat 5 to 7 minutes per side or until no longer pink in center. Cool slightly; cut into thin strips.

3. Arrange lettuce on serving plates. Top with chicken, tomato, bacon and egg. Serve with additional mayonnaise, if desired.

Chicken Salad Bowl

MAKES 4 SERVINGS

CHICKEN

- 3 tablespoons olive oil, divided
- 1 teaspoon salt
- 1 teaspoon dried oregano
- 1 teaspoon paprika
- ½ teaspoon black pepper
- 1 clove garlic, minced
- 1 pound chicken tenders, cut in half

SALAD AND DRESSING

- ⅓ cup olive oil
- 3 tablespoons red wine vinegar
- 1 clove garlic, minced
  Salt and black pepper
- 1 cup grape tomatoes, halved
- 1 cucumber, halved crosswise and cut into sticks
- 1 red bell pepper, sliced
- 2 avocados, thinly sliced
- 2 radishes, thinly sliced
  Coarsely chopped leaf lettuce

1. Combine 1 tablespoon oil, 1 teaspoon salt, oregano, paprika, ½ teaspoon black pepper and 1 clove garlic in large bowl. Add chicken; toss until well coated.

2. Heat remaining 2 tablespoons oil in large skillet over medium-high heat. Add chicken; cook 8 to 10 minutes or until no longer pink, turning once.

3. For dressing, whisk ⅓ cup oil, vinegar and 1 clove garlic in small bowl. Season to taste with salt and black pepper.

4. Place tomatoes, cucumber, bell pepper, avocado slices, radishes and lettuce in serving bowls; drizzle with dressing. Slice chicken and place on salads.

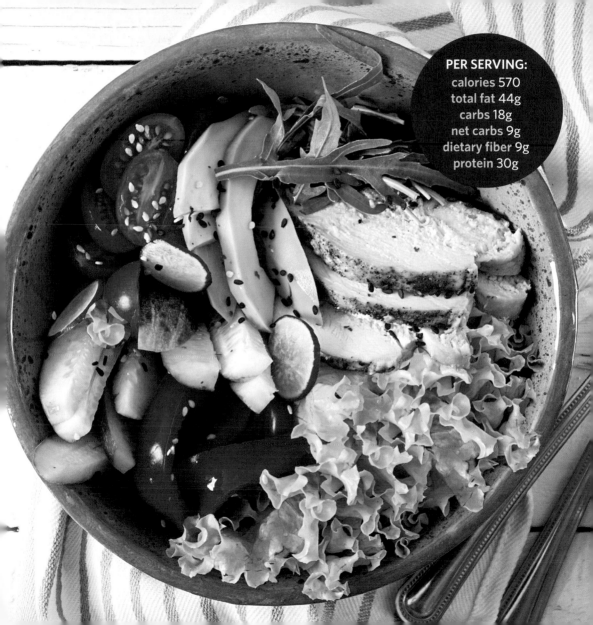

PER SERVING:
calories 570
total fat 44g
carbs 18g
net carbs 9g
dietary fiber 9g
protein 30g

Salmon Salad
with Basil Vinaigrette

MAKES 4 SERVINGS

BASIL VINAIGRETTE

- 3 tablespoons extra virgin olive oil
- 1 tablespoon white wine vinegar
- 1 tablespoon minced fresh basil
- 1 clove garlic, minced
- 1 teaspoon minced fresh chives
- ½ teaspoon salt
- ¼ teaspoon black pepper

SALAD

- 1¼ teaspoons salt, divided
- 1 pound asparagus, trimmed
- 1 pound salmon fillet
- 1½ teaspoons olive oil
- ¼ teaspoon black pepper
- 4 lemon wedges

1. For vinaigrette, whisk 3 tablespoons oil, vinegar, basil, garlic, chives, ½ teaspoon salt and ¼ teaspoon pepper in small bowl until well blended.

2. Preheat oven to 400°F or prepare grill for direct cooking. Place 3 inches of water and 1 teaspoon salt in large saucepan; bring to a boil over high heat. Add asparagus; simmer 6 to 8 minutes or until crisp-tender; drain and set aside.

3. Brush salmon with 1½ teaspoons oil. Sprinkle with remaining ¼ teaspoon salt and ¼ teaspoon pepper. Place fish in shallow baking pan; cook 11 to 13 minutes or until center is opaque. (Or grill on well-oiled grid over medium-high heat 4 or 5 minutes per side or until center is opaque.)

4. Remove skin from salmon; break into bite-size pieces. Arrange salmon over asparagus; drizzle with vinaigrette. Serve with lemon wedges.

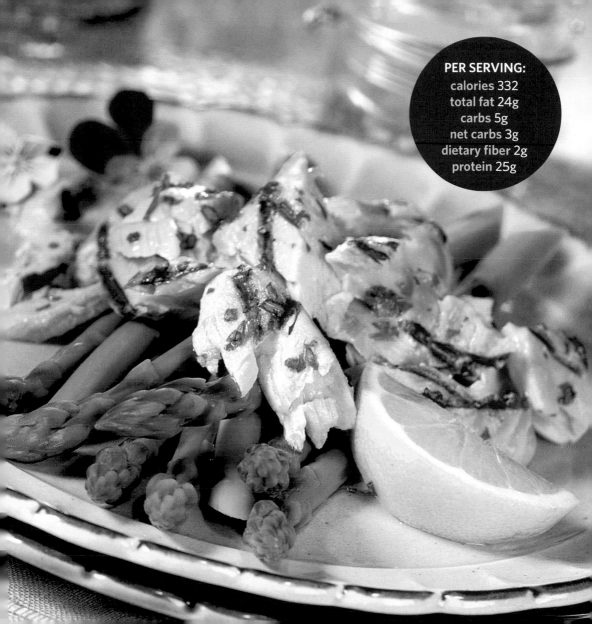

PER SERVING:
calories 332
total fat 24g
carbs 5g
net carbs 3g
dietary fiber 2g
protein 25g

Spiced Chicken Skewers with Yogurt-Tahini Sauce

MAKES 8 SERVINGS

1 cup plain nonfat or regular Greek yogurt

¼ cup chopped fresh parsley, plus additional for garnish

¼ cup tahini

2 tablespoons lemon juice

1 clove garlic

¾ teaspoon salt, divided

1 tablespoon vegetable oil

2 teaspoons garam masala

1 pound boneless skinless chicken breasts, cut into 1-inch pieces

1. Spray grid with nonstick cooking spray. Prepare grill for direct cooking.

2. For sauce, combine yogurt, ¼ cup parsley, tahini, lemon juice, garlic and ¼ teaspoon salt in food processor or blender; process until smooth. Set aside.

3. Combine oil, garam masala and remaining ½ teaspoon salt in medium bowl. Add chicken; toss to coat. Thread chicken on 8 (6-inch) wooden or metal skewers.

4. Grill chicken skewers over medium-high heat 5 minutes per side or until chicken is no longer pink. Serve with sauce. Garnish with additional parsley.

VARIATION: To broil chicken, place skewers on baking sheet or in 13×9-inch baking pan. Broil skewers 10 to 15 minutes or until chicken is cooked through.

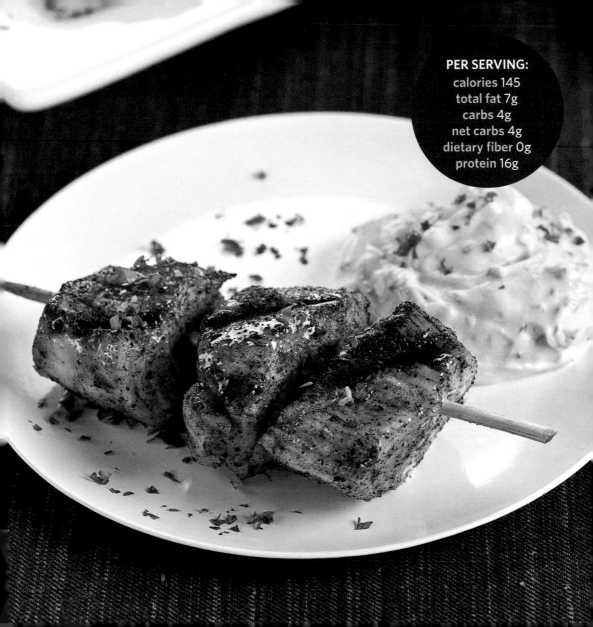

PER SERVING:
calories 145
total fat 7g
carbs 4g
net carbs 4g
dietary fiber 0g
protein 16g

Market Salad

MAKES 4 SERVINGS

3 eggs
4 cups mixed baby salad greens
2 cups green beans, cut into
    1½-inch pieces, cooked and
    drained
4 slices thick-cut bacon, crisp-
    cooked and crumbled

1 tablespoon minced fresh basil,
    chives or Italian parsley
3 tablespoons olive oil
1 tablespoon red wine vinegar
1 teaspoon Dijon mustard
¼ teaspoon salt
¼ teaspoon black pepper

1. Bring medium saucepan of water to a boil. Gently add eggs with slotted spoon. Reduce heat to maintain a simmer; cook 12 minutes. Meanwhile, fill medium bowl with cold water and ice cubes. Drain eggs and place in ice water; cool 10 minutes.

2. Combine salad greens, green beans, bacon and basil in large serving bowl. Peel and coarsely chop eggs; add to serving bowl. Whisk oil, vinegar, mustard, salt and pepper in small bowl until well blended. Drizzle dressing over salad; toss gently to coat.

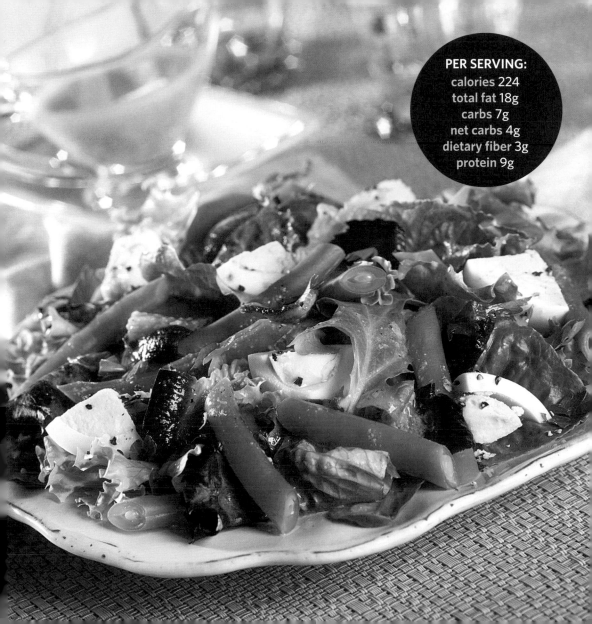

PER SERVING:
calories 224
total fat 18g
carbs 7g
net carbs 4g
dietary fiber 3g
protein 9g

Veggie-Packed Pizza

MAKES 6 SERVINGS

2½ cups finely chopped fresh cauliflower (about ½ head)*

1½ cups (6 ounces) shredded mozzarella cheese, divided

1 egg

4 teaspoons chopped fresh oregano, divided

½ cup sliced mushrooms

½ cup sliced bell pepper (red, yellow, green or a combination)

½ cup sliced red onion

2 teaspoons olive oil

3 tablespoons pizza sauce

Dash red pepper flakes

To chop cauliflower easily, place in food processor and pulse until finely chopped.

1. Preheat oven to 450°F. Spray pizza pan with nonstick cooking spray. Line large baking sheet with foil.

2. Place cauliflower in medium microwavable bowl; microwave on HIGH 4 minutes. Stir; microwave on HIGH 4 minutes or until tender. Let cool slightly.

3. Add 1 cup cheese, egg and 2 teaspoons oregano to cauliflower; mix well. Pat mixture into 9-inch circle in prepared pizza pan; spray with cooking spray.

4. Combine mushrooms, bell peppers and onion on prepared baking sheet. Drizzle with oil; toss to coat.

5. Roast vegetables 14 to 15 minutes or until tender. Bake cauliflower crust during last 10 to 12 minutes of cooking time or until crust is golden brown around edges.

6. Spread pizza sauce over crust; top with roasted vegetables and remaining ½ cup cheese. Bake 6 to 7 minutes or just until cheese is melted. Sprinkle with remaining 2 teaspoons oregano and red pepper flakes. Cut into 6 wedges.

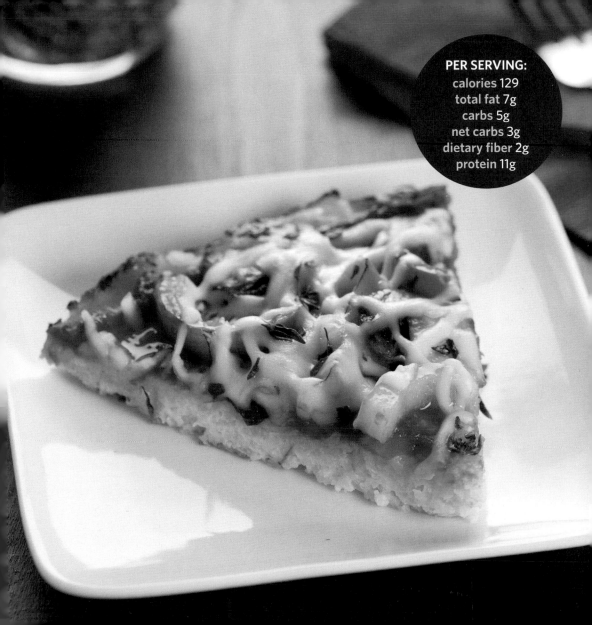

PER SERVING:
calories 129
total fat 7g
carbs 5g
net carbs 3g
dietary fiber 2g
protein 11g

Mini Spinach Frittatas

MAKES 12 MINI FRITTATAS (4 PER SERVING)

1 tablespoon olive oil

½ cup chopped onion

8 eggs

¼ cup plain yogurt

1 package (10 ounces) frozen chopped spinach, thawed and squeezed dry

½ cup (2 ounces) shredded white Cheddar cheese

¼ cup grated Parmesan cheese

¾ teaspoon salt

⅛ teaspoon black pepper

⅛ teaspoon ground red pepper

Dash ground nutmeg

1. Preheat oven to 350°F. Spray 12 standard (2½-inch) muffin cups with nonstick cooking spray.

2. Heat oil in large nonstick skillet over medium heat. Add onion; cook and stir about 5 minutes or until tender. Set aside to cool slightly.

3. Whisk eggs and yogurt in large bowl. Stir in spinach, Cheddar, Parmesan, salt, black pepper, red pepper, nutmeg and onion until blended. Divide mixture evenly among prepared muffin cups.

4. Bake 20 to 25 minutes or until eggs are puffed and firm and no longer shiny. Cool in pan 2 minutes. Loosen bottom and sides with small spatula or knife; remove to wire rack. Serve warm, cold or at room temperature.

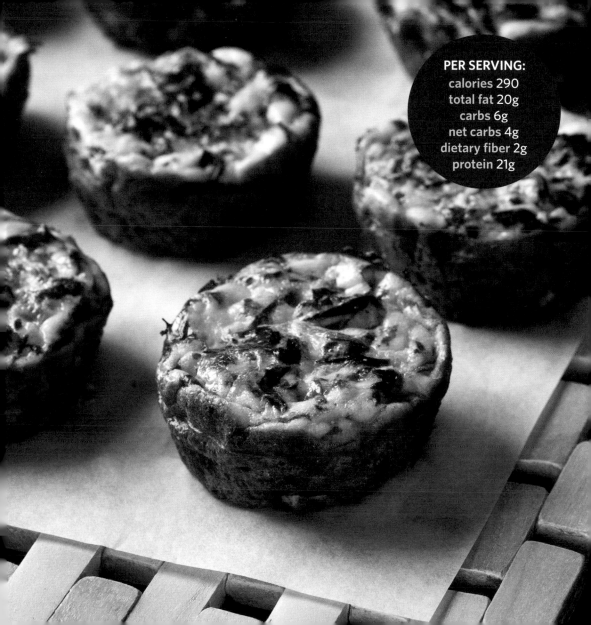

PER SERVING:
calories 290
total fat 20g
carbs 6g
net carbs 4g
dietary fiber 2g
protein 21g

Smoked Salmon Omelet Roll-Ups

MAKES ABOUT 24 PIECES

4 eggs
⅛ teaspoon black pepper
¼ cup plain or chive and onion cream cheese, softened

1 package (about 4 ounces) smoked salmon, cut into bite-size pieces

1. Beat eggs and pepper in small bowl until well blended (no streaks of white showing). Spray large nonstick skillet with nonstick cooking spray; heat over medium-high heat.

2. Pour half of egg mixture into skillet; tilt skillet to completely coat bottom with thin layer of eggs. Cook 2 to 4 minutes without stirring or until eggs are set. Use spatula to carefully loosen omelet from skillet; slide onto cutting board. Repeat with remaining egg mixture to make second omelet.

3. Spread 2 tablespoons cream cheese over each omelet; top with smoked salmon pieces. Tightly roll up omelets; wrap in plastic wrap and refrigerate at least 30 minutes. Cut off ends, then cut rolls crosswise into ½-inch slices.

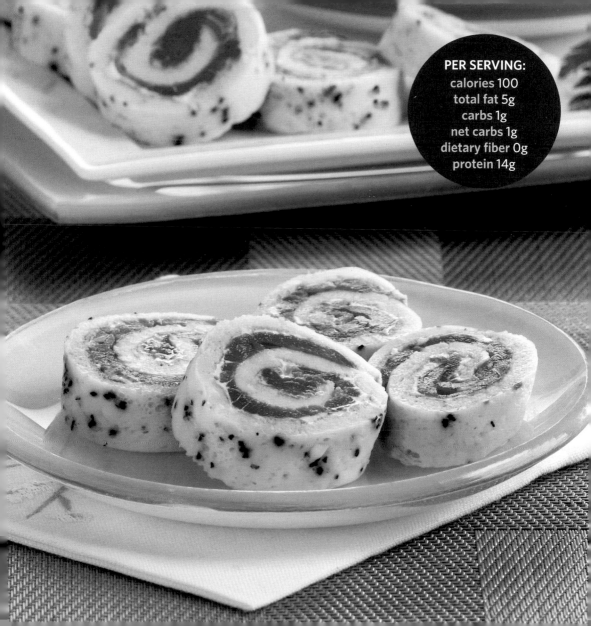

PER SERVING:
calories 100
total fat 5g
carbs 1g
net carbs 1g
dietary fiber 0g
protein 14g

Spicy Chicken Bundles

MAKES 12 BUNDLES

1 pound ground chicken or
    turkey

2 teaspoons minced fresh ginger

2 cloves garlic, minced

¼ teaspoon red pepper flakes

1 tablespoon peanut oil

3 tablespoons soy sauce

⅓ cup finely chopped water
    chestnuts

⅓ cup thinly sliced green onions

¼ cup chopped peanuts

12 large lettuce leaves, such as
    romaine

   Whole fresh chives (optional)

   Chinese hot mustard (optional)

1. Combine chicken, ginger, garlic and red pepper flakes in medium bowl.

2. Heat oil in wok or large skillet over medium-high heat. Add chicken mixture; stir-fry 2 to 3 minutes until chicken is cooked through.

3. Add soy sauce; cook and stir 30 seconds. Add water chestnuts, green onions and peanuts; heat through.

4. Divide filling evenly among lettuce leaves; roll up and secure with chives or toothpicks. Serve warm or at room temperature. Do not let filling stand at room temperature more than 2 hours. Serve with hot mustard, if desired.

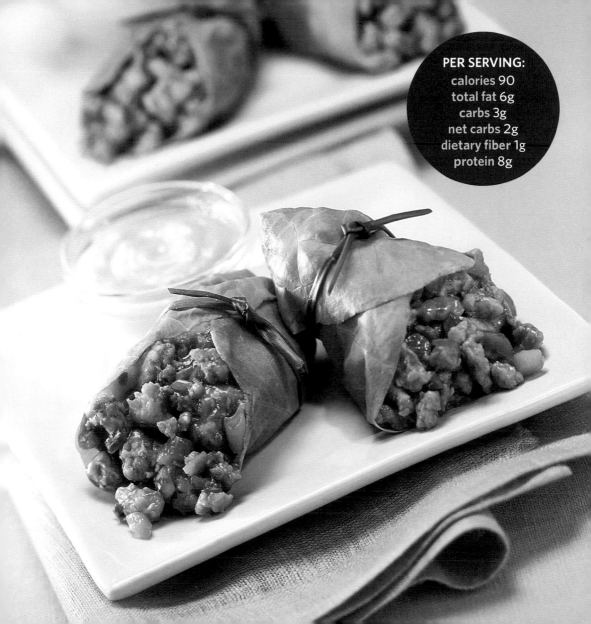

Ham and Cheese Rolls

MAKES 8 SERVINGS (64 PIECES)

4 thin slices deli ham (about 4×4 inches)

1 package (8 ounces) cream cheese, softened

1 piece (4 inches long) seedless cucumber, quartered lengthwise (about ½ cucumber)

4 thin slices (about 4×4 inches) American or Cheddar cheese, at room temperature

1 red bell pepper, cut into thin 4-inch-long strips

1. For ham sushi, pat 1 ham slice with paper towel to remove excess moisture and place on cutting board. Spread 2 tablespoons cream cheese to edges of ham slice. Pat 1 cucumber piece with paper towel to remove excess moisture; place at edge of ham slice. Roll up tightly, pressing gently to seal. Wrap in plastic wrap; refrigerate. Repeat with remaining ham slices, cream cheese and cucumber pieces.

2. For cheese sushi, spread 2 tablespoons cream cheese to edges of 1 cheese slice. Place 2 red pepper strips at edge of cheese slice. Roll up tightly, pressing gently to seal. Wrap in plastic wrap; refrigerate. Repeat with remaining cheese slices, cream cheese and red pepper strips.

3. To serve, remove plastic wrap from ham and cheese rolls. Cut each roll into ½-inch pieces.

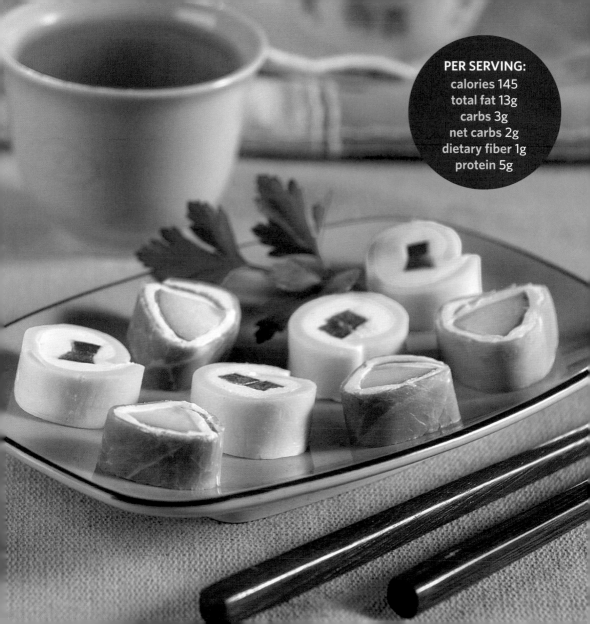

PER SERVING:
calories 145
total fat 13g
carbs 3g
net carbs 2g
dietary fiber 1g
protein 5g

Tuna Melt

MAKES 4 SERVINGS

¾ cup mayonnaise

2 teaspoons lemon juice

1 teaspoon salt

⅛ teaspoon black pepper

1 can (12 ounces) solid white albacore tuna, drained

1 can (12 ounces) chunk light tuna, drained

1 stalk celery, finely chopped (about ½ cup)

¼ cup minced red onion

½ loaf keto bread (page 138), cut into 8 slices

8 slices Cheddar cheese

2 tablespoons butter

Optional toppings: tomato slices, onion slices, pickles, sliced avocado and/or lettuce leaves

1. Combine mayonnaise, lemon juice, salt and pepper in large bowl. Add tuna, celery and red onion; mix well.

2. Divide tuna among bread slices; top each with cheese. Heat 1 tablespoon butter in large skillet over medium heat until melted. Add half of sandwiches; cover and cook until bread is toasted and cheese is melted. Repeat with remaining butter and sandwiches. Garnish with desired toppings.

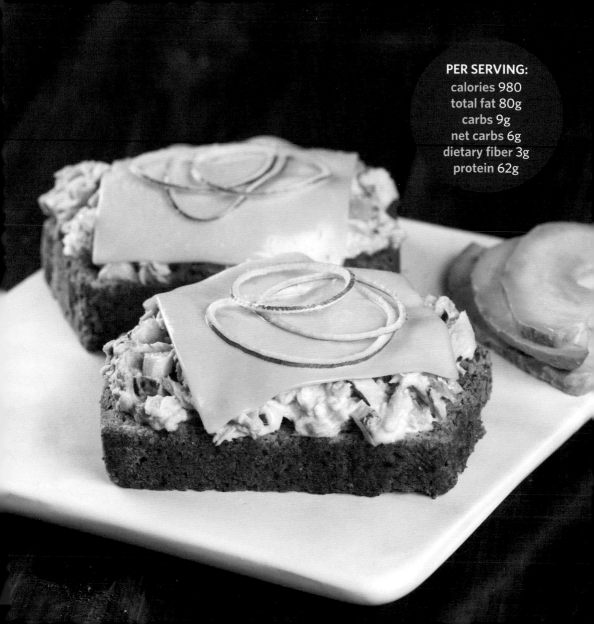

PER SERVING:
calories 980
total fat 80g
carbs 9g
net carbs 6g
dietary fiber 3g
protein 62g

Asparagus Roll-Ups

MAKES ABOUT 24 ROLL-UPS

1 **pound asparagus, tough ends trimmed (about 24 spears)**

½ **(8-ounce) package cream cheese, softened**

½ **pound thinly sliced salami**

1. Cut asparagus into lengths 1 inch longer than width of salami. Reserve bottoms for another use. Simmer asparagus in salted water in large skillet 4 to 5 minutes or until crisp-tender. Drain; immediately immerse in cold water to stop cooking. Drain; pat dry with paper towel.

2. Spread about 1 teaspoon cream cheese evenly over one side of each salami slice. Roll up 1 asparagus spear with each salami slice.

3. Cover and refrigerate. Let stand at room temperature 10 minutes before serving.

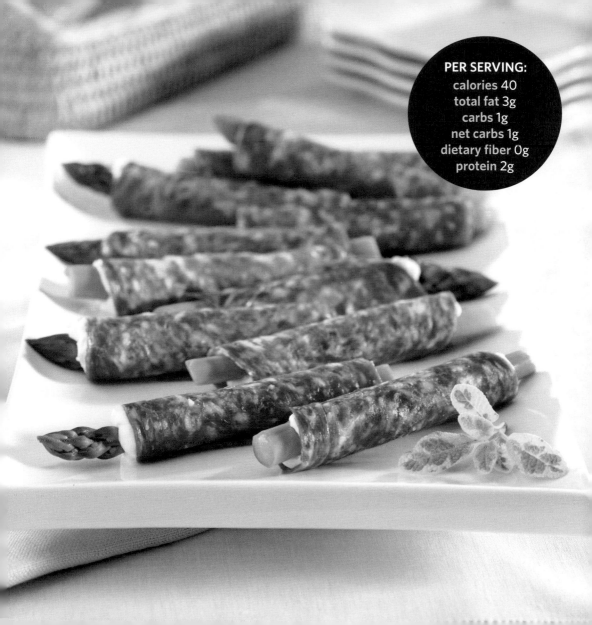

PER SERVING:
calories 40
total fat 3g
carbs 1g
net carbs 1g
dietary fiber 0g
protein 2g

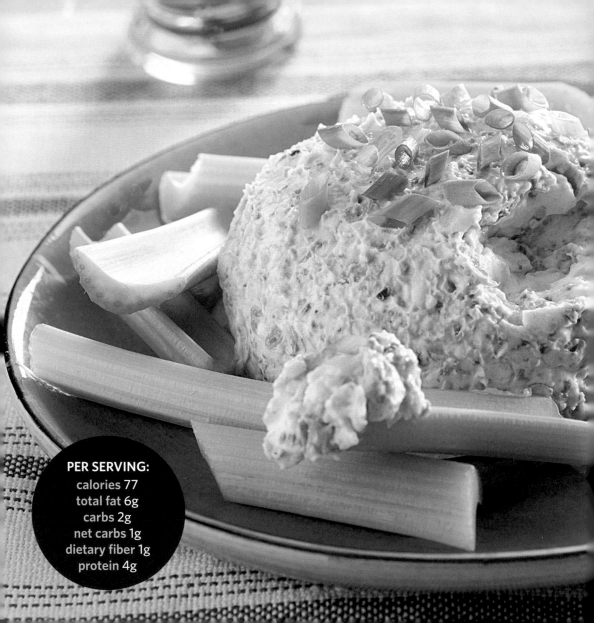

PER SERVING:
calories 77
total fat 6g
carbs 2g
net carbs 1g
dietary fiber 1g
protein 4g

Snacks

Bacon and Onion Cheese Ball

MAKES 2½ CUPS (2 TABLESPOONS PER SERVING)

1 package (8 ounces) cream
   cheese, softened
½ cup sour cream
½ cup chopped cooked bacon

½ cup chopped green onions,
   plus additional for garnish
¼ cup crumbled blue cheese
Celery sticks (optional)

1. Beat cream cheese, sour cream, bacon, ½ cup green onions and blue cheese in large bowl until well blended. Shape mixture into a ball. Wrap in plastic wrap; refrigerate at least 1 hour.

2. Place cheese ball on serving plate. Garnish with additional green onions. Serve with celery, if desired.

Prosciutto-Wrapped Asparagus with Garlic Mayonnaise

MAKES 8 SERVINGS

- **2 tablespoons olive oil, divided**
- **1 package (about 3 ounces) prosciutto, cut lengthwise into 16 strips**
- **16 medium asparagus spears, trimmed**
- **Black pepper (optional)**
- **3/4 cup mayonnaise**
- **1 teaspoon lemon juice**
- **1 clove garlic, minced**

1. Preheat oven to 400°F. Brush large shallow baking pan with 1 tablespoon oil. Wrap 1 piece of prosciutto around each asparagus spear. Place asparagus on prepared baking pan. Brush asparagus with remaining oil; sprinkle with pepper, if desired.

2. Bake about 12 minutes or until asparagus is tender. Cool slightly.

3. Meanwhile for garlic mayonnaise, combine mayonnaise, lemon juice and garlic in small bowl until well blended. Serve with warm asparagus.

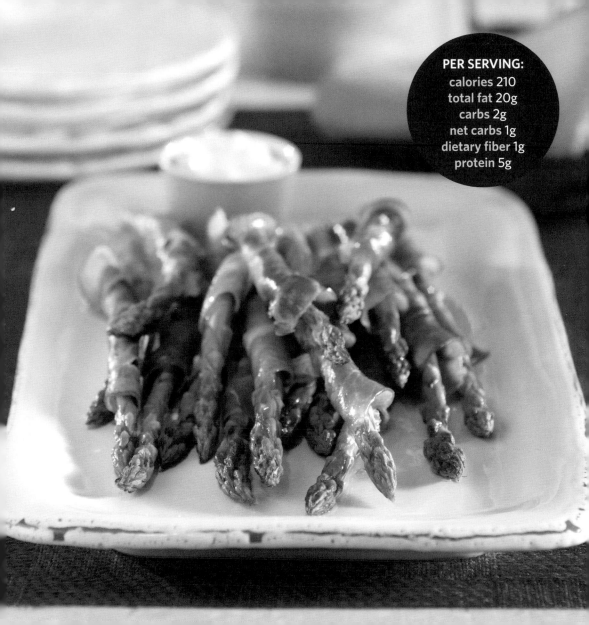

PER SERVING:
calories 210
total fat 20g
carbs 2g
net carbs 1g
dietary fiber 1g
protein 5g

Smoked Salmon Spread

MAKES 1½ CUPS (2 TABLESPOONS PER SERVING)

1 package (8 ounces) cream cheese, softened

3 ounces smoked salmon, coarsely chopped

2 tablespoons fresh lemon juice

1 tablespoon chopped fresh dill

1 tablespoon capers

Cucumber slices

1. Combine cream cheese, salmon, lemon juice, dill and capers in small bowl; mix well.

2. Serve immediately or cover and refrigerate up to 24 hours. Serve with cucumber slices.

TIP: This savory spread can be prepared up to 3 days in advance, covered with plastic wrap and refrigerated.

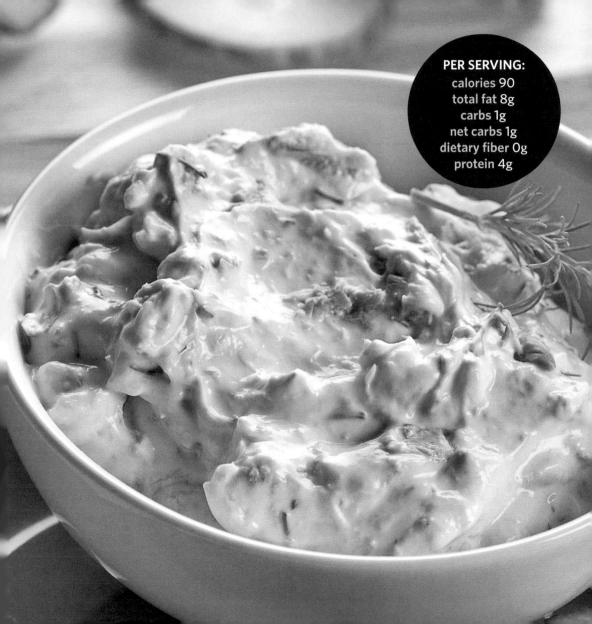

PER SERVING:
calories 90
total fat 8g
carbs 1g
net carbs 1g
dietary fiber 0g
protein 4g

Mini Spinach and Bacon Quiches

MAKES 12 SERVINGS

3 slices bacon

½ small onion, diced

1 package (10 ounces) frozen chopped spinach, thawed and squeezed dry

½ teaspoon black pepper

⅛ teaspoon ground nutmeg

Pinch salt

3 eggs

1 container (15 ounces) whole-milk ricotta cheese

2 cups (8 ounces) shredded mozzarella cheese

1 cup grated Parmesan cheese

1. Preheat oven to 350°F. Spray 12 standard (2½-inch) muffin cups with nonstick cooking spray.

2. Cook bacon in large skillet until crisp. Drain on paper towels. Crumble when cool enough to handle.

3. Heat same skillet with bacon drippings over medium heat. Add onion; cook and stir 5 minutes or until tender. Add spinach, pepper, nutmeg and salt; cook and stir 3 minutes or until liquid is evaporated. Remove from heat. Stir in bacon; set aside to cool.

4. Whisk eggs in large bowl. Add cheeses; stir until well blended. Add cooled spinach mixture; mix well. Spoon evenly into prepared muffin cups.

5. Bake 40 minutes or until set. Cool in pan 10 minutes. Run thin knife around edges to remove from pan. Serve immediately.

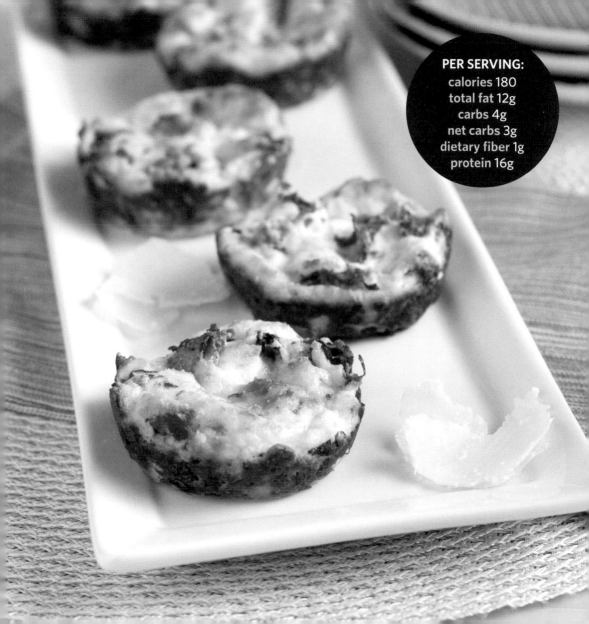

PER SERVING:
calories 180
total fat 12g
carbs 4g
net carbs 3g
dietary fiber 1g
protein 16g

Shrimp Pâté

MAKES 1½ CUPS SPREAD (2 TABLESPOONS PER SERVING)

- 8 ounces cooked peeled shrimp
- ¼ cup (½ stick) butter, cut into chunks
- 2 teaspoons dry vermouth or chicken broth
- 1 teaspoon lemon juice
- 1 teaspoon Dijon mustard
- ¼ teaspoon salt
- ¼ teaspoon ground mace
- ⅛ teaspoon ground red pepper
- ⅛ teaspoon black pepper
- ½ cup chopped shelled pistachios
- 2 large heads Belgian endive

1. Combine shrimp, butter, vermouth, lemon juice, mustard, salt, mace, red pepper and black pepper in blender or food processor. Process until smooth. Shape mixture into 8-inch log on waxed paper. (If mixture is too soft to handle refrigerate 1 hour.)

2. Spread pistachios on sheet of waxed paper. Roll pâté log in nuts to coat. Cover and refrigerate 1 to 3 hours.

3. Separate endive into individual leaves. Place pâté on serving plate; serve with endive leaves.

VARIATION: Spoon shrimp pâté into serving bowl and sprinkle with pistachio nuts.

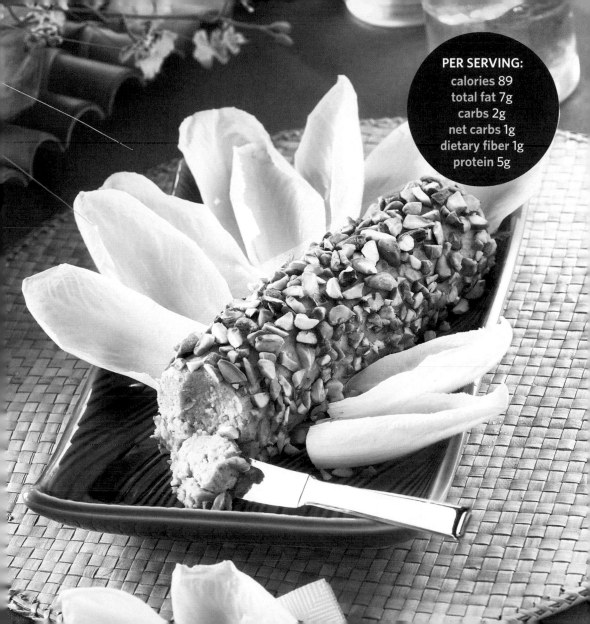

PER SERVING:
calories 89
total fat 7g
carbs 2g
net carbs 1g
dietary fiber 1g
protein 5g

Rosemary Nut Mix

2 **tablespoons butter**
2 **cups pecan halves**
1 **cup unsalted macadamia nuts**
1 **cup walnuts**

1 **teaspoon dried rosemary**
½ **teaspoon salt**
¼ **teaspoon red pepper flakes**

1. Preheat oven to 300°F.

2. Melt butter in large saucepan over low heat. Stir in pecans, macadamia nuts and walnuts. Add rosemary, salt and red pepper flakes; cook and stir about 1 minute. Spread mixture on ungreased baking sheet.

3. Bake 8 to 10 minutes, stirring occasionally. Cool completely on baking sheet on wire rack.

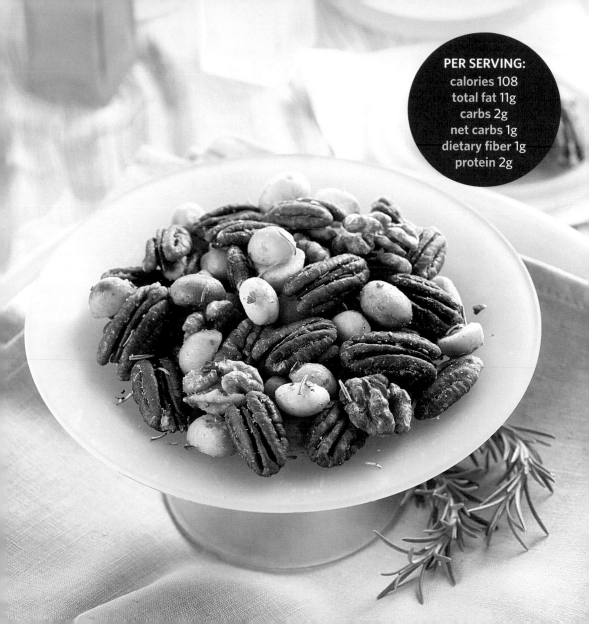

PER SERVING:
calories 108
total fat 11g
carbs 2g
net carbs 1g
dietary fiber 1g
protein 2g

Zucchini Pizza Bites

MAKES 8 SERVINGS

1 medium zucchini

3 tablespoons pizza sauce

2 tablespoons tomato paste

¼ teaspoon dried oregano

¾ cup (3 ounces) shredded
mozzarella cheese

¼ cup shredded Parmesan cheese

8 slices pitted black olives

8 slices pepperoni

1. Preheat broiler; set rack 4 inches from heat.

2. Trim and discard ends of zucchini. Cut zucchini into 16 (¼-inch-thick) diagonal slices. Place on nonstick baking sheet.

3. Combine pizza sauce, tomato paste and oregano in small bowl; mix well. Spread scant teaspoon sauce over each zucchini slice. Combine cheeses in small bowl. Top each zucchini slice with 1 tablespoon cheese mixture, pressing down into sauce. Place 1 olive slice on each of 8 pizza bites. Place 1 folded pepperoni slice on each remaining pizza bite.

4. Broil 3 minutes or until cheese is melted. Serve immediately.

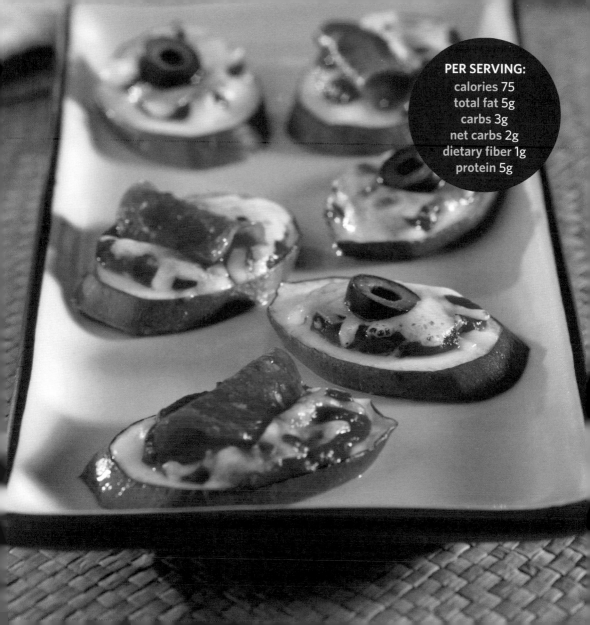

PER SERVING:
calories 75
total fat 5g
carbs 3g
net carbs 2g
dietary fiber 1g
protein 5g

Parmesan-Pepper Crisps

MAKES ABOUT 26 CRISPS

2   **cups loosely packed coarsely grated Parmesan cheese**

2   **teaspoons black pepper**

1. Preheat oven to 400°F. Line wire racks with paper towels.

2. Place heaping teaspoonfuls of cheese 2 inches apart on ungreased nonstick baking sheet. Flatten cheese mounds slightly with back of spoon. Sprinkle each with pepper.

3. Bake 15 to 20 minutes or until crisps are very lightly browned. (Watch closely—crisps burn easily.) Cool 2 minutes on baking sheet. Carefully remove with spatula to prepared racks. Store in airtight container in refrigerator up to 3 days.

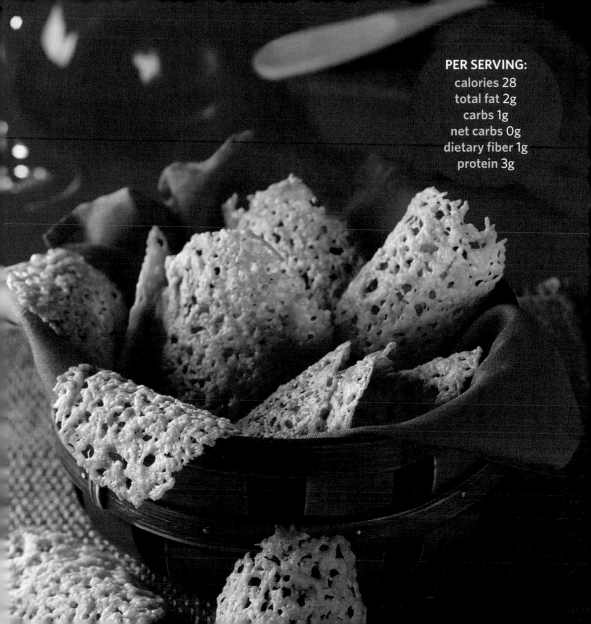

PER SERVING:
calories 28
total fat 2g
carbs 1g
net carbs 0g
dietary fiber 1g
protein 3g

Avocado Salsa

MAKES ABOUT 4 CUPS (2 TABLESPOONS PER SERVING)

1 medium avocado, diced

1 cup chopped onion

1 cup peeled seeded chopped cucumber

1 Anaheim pepper, seeded and chopped

½ cup chopped fresh tomato

2 tablespoons chopped fresh cilantro

½ teaspoon salt

¼ teaspoon hot pepper sauce

Combine avocado, onion, cucumber, Anaheim pepper, tomato, 2 tablespoons cilantro, salt and hot pepper sauce in medium bowl; mix gently. Cover and refrigerate at least 1 hour before serving.

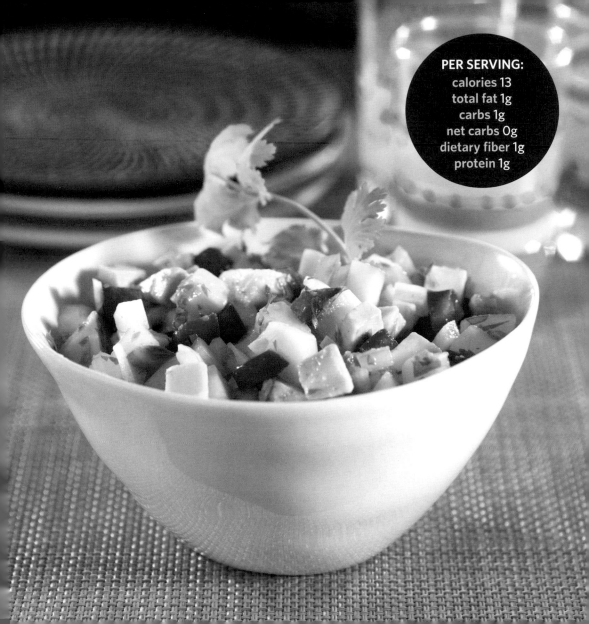

PER SERVING:
calories 13
total fat 1g
carbs 1g
net carbs 0g
dietary fiber 1g
protein 1g

Picante Vegetable Dip

MAKES ABOUT 1⅔ CUPS (2 TABLESPOONS PER SERVING)

⅔ cup reduced-fat or regular sour
   cream

½ cup picante sauce

⅓ cup mayonnaise

¼ cup finely chopped green or
   red bell pepper

2 tablespoons finely chopped
   green onion

¾ teaspoon garlic salt
   Cut-up fresh vegetables

Combine sour cream, picante sauce, mayonnaise, bell pepper, green onion and garlic salt in medium bowl until well blended. Cover; refrigerate several hours or overnight to allow flavors to blend. Serve with vegetables for dipping.

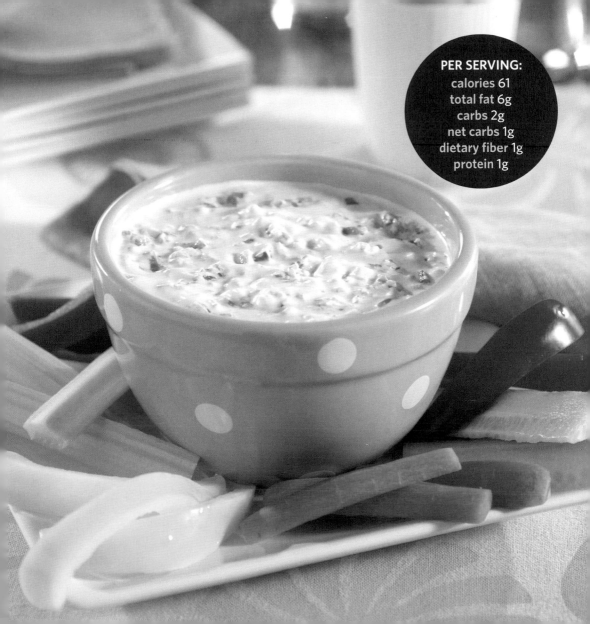

PER SERVING:
calories 61
total fat 6g
carbs 2g
net carbs 1g
dietary fiber 1g
protein 1g

Crispy Mozzarella Chips

MAKES 8 SERVINGS

1½ **cups (6 ounces) shredded**
    mozzarella cheese*

½ **cup grated Parmesan cheese**

4 **green onions**

1 **teaspoon chili powder**

1 **teaspoon black pepper**

*Shred cheese using largest holes on box
grater. If purchasing shredded cheese, look
for "chef-style" cheese which is grated into
larger than usual pieces.*

1. Place mozzarella cheese in colander with large holes; shake to separate large shreds of cheese from smaller shreds; save smaller shreds for another use. Transfer large shreds of cheese to medium bowl; add Parmesan and toss to blend.

2. Remove white ends from green onions. Slit open onions lengthwise with paring knife and then thinly slice crosswise. Add to bowl with cheeses. Add chili powder and pepper; toss gently.

3. Spray medium nonstick skillet with nonstick cooking spray; heat over medium-high heat. Sprinkle about 1 tablespoon cheese mixture in single layer in skillet making lacy 2-inch circle. Cook 1 to 1½ minutes until cheese melts and turns golden brown. Immediately remove from skillet with thin spatula; cool completely on parchment-lined baking sheet. Repeat with remaining cheese mixture.

NOTE: Cheese crisps are extremely hot and pliable when they are first removed from the skillet but become crispy and chewy as they cool. You can easily mold them by draping them over a rolling pin.

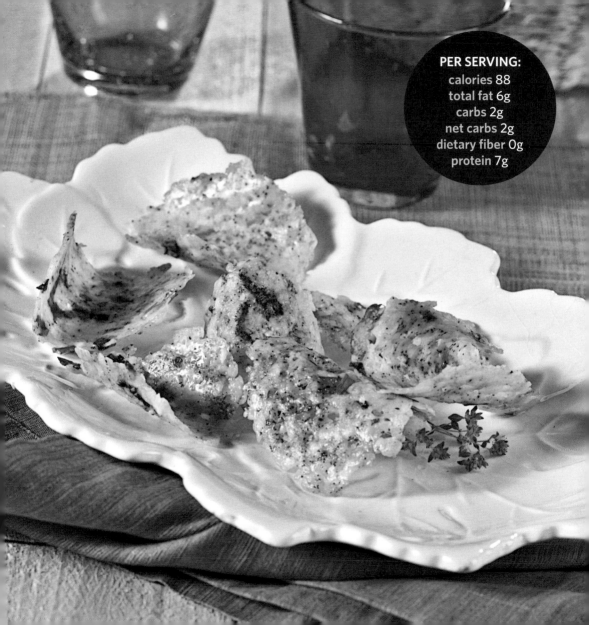

PER SERVING:
calories 88
total fat 6g
carbs 2g
net carbs 2g
dietary fiber 0g
protein 7g

Bacon and Cheese Dip

MAKES ABOUT 4 CUPS (¼ CUP PER SERVING)

- 2 packages (8 ounces each) cream cheese, cut into cubes
- 4 cups (16 ounces) shredded Colby-Jack cheese
- 1 cup whipping cream
- 2 tablespoons prepared mustard
- 1 tablespoon minced onion
- 2 teaspoons Worcestershire sauce
- ½ teaspoon salt
- ¼ teaspoon hot pepper sauce
- 1 pound bacon, crisp-cooked and crumbled

Cut-up fresh vegetables

SLOW COOKER DIRECTIONS

1. Combine cream cheese, Colby-Jack cheese, cream, mustard, onion, Worcestershire sauce, salt and hot pepper sauce in 1½-quart slow cooker.

2. Cover; cook on LOW 1 hour or until cheeses are melted, stirring occasionally.

3. Stir in bacon; adjust seasonings. Serve with vegetables.

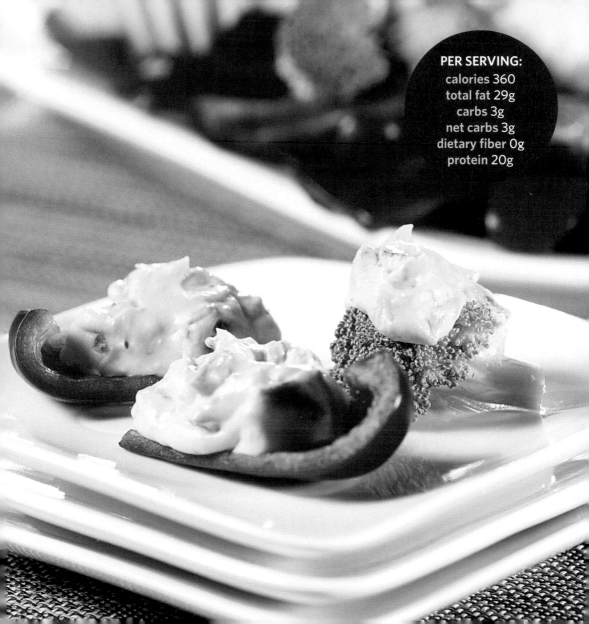

PER SERVING:
calories 360
total fat 29g
carbs 3g
net carbs 3g
dietary fiber 0g
protein 20g

Grilled Feta with Peppers

MAKES 8 SERVINGS

¼ **cup thinly sliced sweet onion**
1 **package (8 ounces) feta cheese, thickly sliced crosswise**
¼ **cup thinly sliced green bell pepper**

¼ **cup thinly sliced red bell pepper**
½ **teaspoon dried oregano**
¼ **teaspoon garlic pepper or black pepper**

1. Spray 14-inch-long sheet of foil with nonstick cooking spray. Place onion in center of foil and top with feta and bell peppers. Sprinkle with oregano and garlic pepper.

2. Bring two long sides of foil together above the food; fold down in a series of locked folds, allowing for heat circulation and expansion. Fold short ends up and over again. Press folds firmly to seal packet. Place foil packet upside down on grid. Grill, covered, over high heat 15 minutes. Turn packet over; grill, covered, 15 minutes.

3. Open packet carefully and serve immediately.

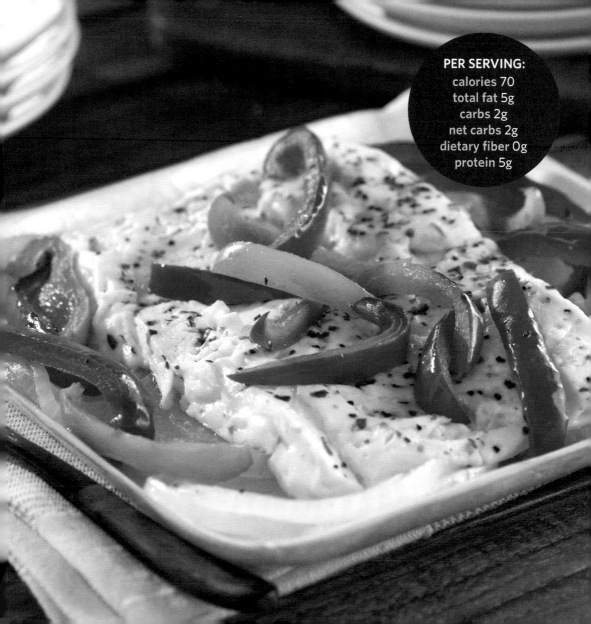

PER SERVING:
calories 70
total fat 5g
carbs 2g
net carbs 2g
dietary fiber 0g
protein 5g

Classic Deviled Eggs

MAKES 12 DEVILED EGGS

 6 **eggs**
 3 **tablespoons mayonnaise**
 ½ **teaspoon apple cider vinegar**
 ½ **teaspoon yellow mustard**
 ⅛ **teaspoon salt**

Optional toppings: black pepper, smoked or regular paprika, chopped fresh dill, minced fresh chives and/or minced red onion (optional)

1. Bring medium saucepan of water to a boil. Gently add eggs with slotted spoon. Reduce heat to maintain a simmer; cook 12 minutes. Meanwhile, fill medium bowl with cold water and ice cubes. Drain eggs and place in ice water; cool 10 minutes.

2. Carefully peel eggs. Cut eggs in half; place yolks in small bowl. Add mayonnaise, vinegar, mustard and salt; mash until well blended. Spoon mixture into egg whites; garnish with desired toppings.

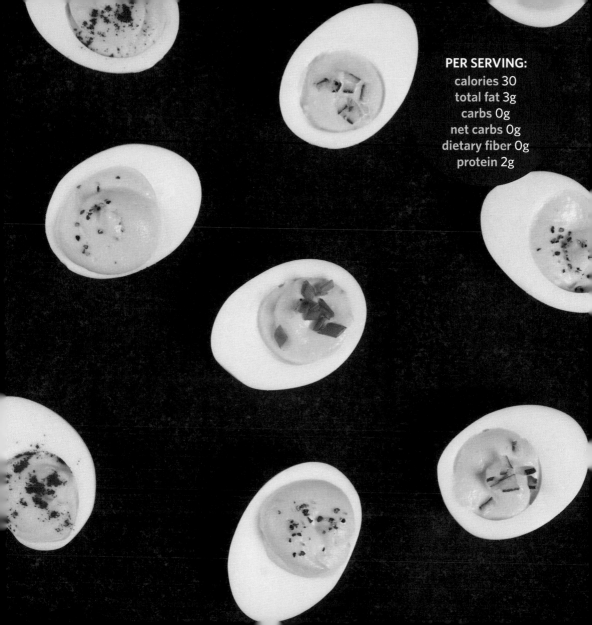

PER SERVING:
calories 30
total fat 3g
carbs 0g
net carbs 0g
dietary fiber 0g
protein 2g

Jalapeño Poppers

MAKES 20 TO 24 POPPERS

10 to 12 fresh jalapeño peppers*

1 package (8 ounces) cream cheese, softened

1½ cups (6 ounces) shredded Cheddar cheese, divided

2 green onions, finely chopped

½ teaspoon onion powder

¼ teaspoon salt

⅛ teaspoon garlic powder

6 slices bacon, crisp-cooked and finely chopped

2 tablespoons almond flour (optional)

2 tablespoons grated Parmesan or Romano cheese

*For large jalapeño peppers, use 10. For small peppers, use 12.

1. Preheat oven to 375°F. Line baking sheet with parchment paper or foil.

2. Cut each pepper in half lengthwise; remove ribs and seeds.

3. Combine cream cheese, 1 cup Cheddar cheese, green onions, onion powder, salt and garlic powder in medium bowl. Stir in bacon. Fill each pepper half with about 1 tablespoon cheese mixture. Place on prepared baking sheet. Sprinkle with remaining ½ cup Cheddar cheese, almond flour, if desired, and Parmesan cheese.

4. Bake 10 to 12 minutes or until cheese is melted but peppers are still firm.

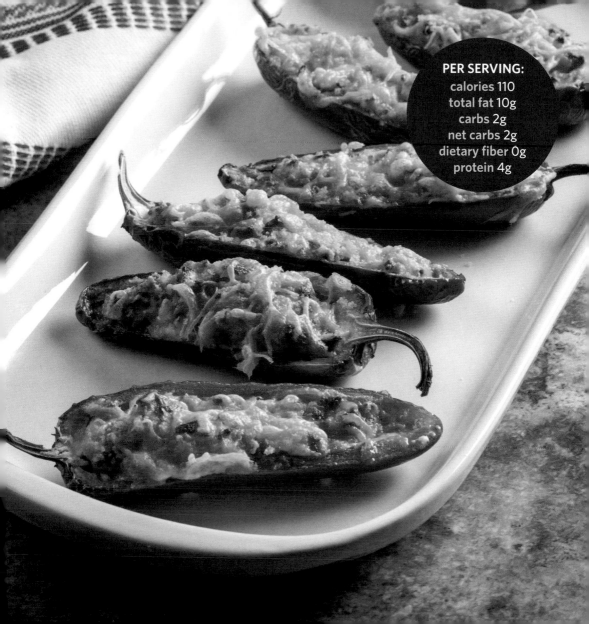

PER SERVING:
calories 110
total fat 10g
carbs 2g
net carbs 2g
dietary fiber 0g
protein 4g

Savory Zucchini Sticks

MAKES 4 SERVINGS (2 STICKS PER SERVING)

6 tablespoons almond flour
¼ cup grated Parmesan cheese
1 egg white
1 tablespoon water

2 small zucchini (about 4 ounces each), cut lengthwise into quarters
⅓ cup pasta sauce, warmed

1. Preheat oven to 400°F. Spray baking sheet with nonstick cooking spray.

2. Combine almond flour and Parmesan in shallow dish. Combine egg white and water in another shallow dish; beat with fork until well blended.

3. Dip each piece of zucchini into egg white mixture, letting excess drip back into dish. Roll in cheese mixture to coat. Place zucchini sticks on prepared baking sheet; spray with nonstick cooking spray.

4. Bake 15 to 18 minutes or until golden brown. Serve with pasta sauce.

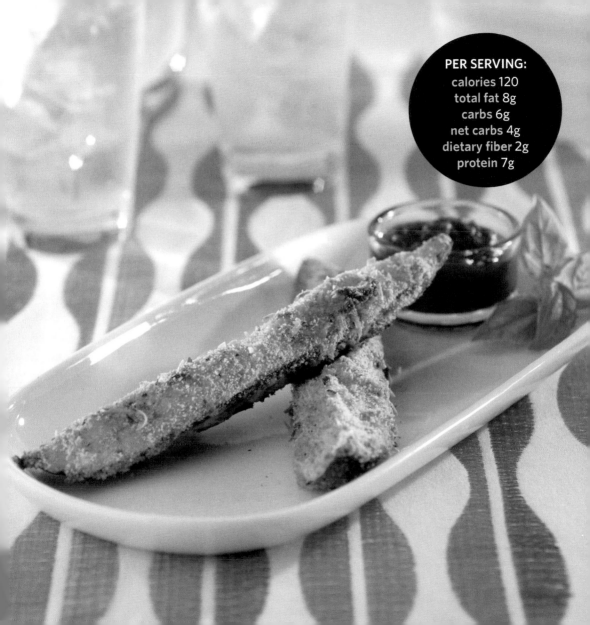

PER SERVING:
calories 120
total fat 8g
carbs 6g
net carbs 4g
dietary fiber 2g
protein 7g

Quick and Easy
Stuffed Mushrooms

MAKES 8 SERVINGS (2 MUSHROOMS PER SERVING)

16 **large mushrooms**
½ **cup sliced celery**
½ **cup sliced onion**
1 **clove garlic**
½ **cup almond flour**

1 **teaspoon Worcestershire sauce**
½ **teaspoon dried marjoram**
⅛ **teaspoon ground red pepper**
Dash paprika

1. Preheat oven to 350°F. Remove stems from mushrooms; reserve caps. Place mushroom stems, celery, onion and garlic in food processor; process using on/off pulses until vegetables are finely chopped.

2. Spray large skillet with nonstick cooking spray. Add vegetable mixture; cook and stir over medium heat 5 minutes or until onion is tender. Remove to bowl. Stir in almond flour, Worcestershire sauce, marjoram and red pepper.

3. Fill mushroom caps evenly with vegetable mixture, pressing down firmly. Place mushrooms about ½ inch apart in shallow baking pan. Spray tops with nonstick cooking spray. Sprinkle with paprika.

4. Bake 15 minutes or until heated through.

NOTE: Mushrooms can be stuffed up to 1 day ahead. Cover and refrigerate until ready to cook. Bake in preheated 300°F oven 20 minutes or until heated through.

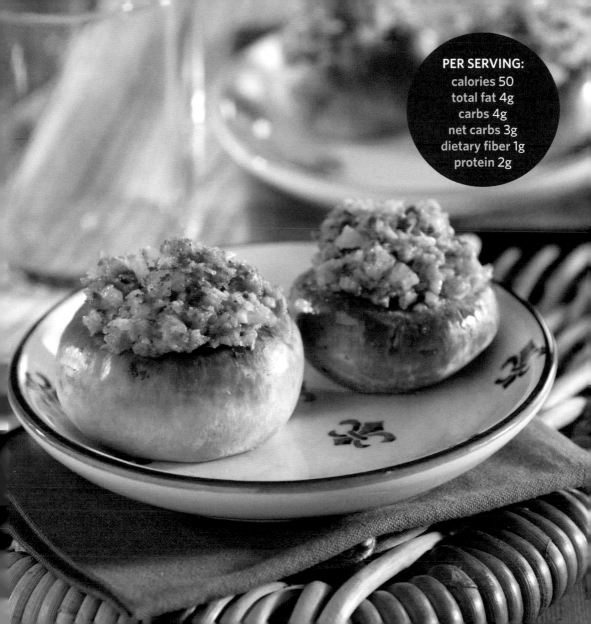

PER SERVING:
calories 50
total fat 4g
carbs 4g
net carbs 3g
dietary fiber 1g
protein 2g

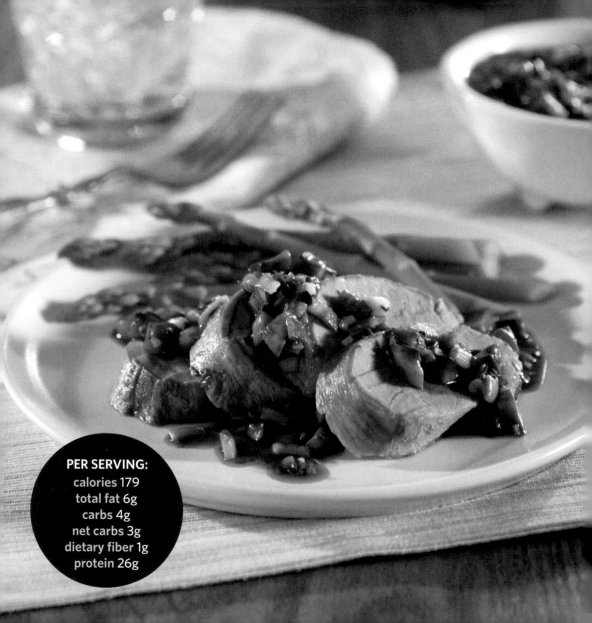

PER SERVING:
calories 179
total fat 6g
carbs 4g
net carbs 3g
dietary fiber 1g
protein 26g

Main Dishes

Pork Tenderloin with Mushroom Sauce

MAKES 4 SERVINGS

1½ pounds pork tenderloin (1 to 2 tenderloins)
Salt and black pepper
1 tablespoon butter
1½ cups chopped button mushrooms or shiitake mushroom caps
2 tablespoons sliced green onion
1 clove garlic, minced
⅓ cup beef broth
1 tablespoon chopped fresh parsley
1 tablespoon dry sherry
½ teaspoon dried thyme

1. Preheat oven to 375°F. Place pork on rack in shallow baking pan; season with salt and pepper. Bake 25 to 35 minutes or until thermometer inserted into thickest part of pork registers 145°F. Let stand, covered, 5 to 10 minutes.

2. Melt butter in medium skillet over medium heat. Add mushrooms, green onion and garlic; cook and stir 3 to 5 minutes or until vegetables are tender. Stir in broth, parsley, sherry and thyme; season with additional salt and pepper. Cook and stir until sauce boils; cook and stir 2 minutes more. Slice pork; serve with sauce.

Greek Lamb with Tzatziki

MAKES 4 SERVINGS

LAMB

- 2½ to 3 pounds boneless leg of lamb
- 4 cloves garlic
- ¼ cup Dijon mustard
- 2 tablespoons minced fresh rosemary leaves
- 2 teaspoons salt
- 2 teaspoons black pepper
- ¼ cup olive oil

TZATZIKI SAUCE

- 4 cloves garlic
- 1 small English cucumber
- 1 tablespoon chopped fresh mint
- 2 teaspoons olive oil
- 1 teaspoon lemon juice
- 2 cups plain Greek yogurt or other thick plain yogurt
- Salt

1. Untie and unroll lamb to lie flat; trim fat.

2. For marinade, mince 4 garlic cloves; place in small bowl. Add mustard, rosemary, 2 teaspoons salt and pepper; whisk in ¼ cup oil. Spread mixture evenly over lamb, coating both sides. Place lamb in large resealable food storage bag. Seal bag; refrigerate at least 2 hours or overnight.

3. Meanwhile for tzatziki sauce, mince 4 garlic cloves and mash to a paste; place in medium bowl. Peel and grate cucumber; squeeze to remove excess moisture. Add cucumber, mint, 2 teaspoons oil and lemon juice to bowl with garlic. Add yogurt; mix well. Season to taste with salt. Refrigerate until ready to serve.

4. Prepare grill for direct cooking. Grill lamb over medium-high heat 35 to 40 minutes or to desired doneness. Cover loosely with foil; let rest 5 to 10 minutes. (Remove from grill at 140°F for medium. Temperature will rise 5°F while resting.) Slice lamb and serve with tzatziki sauce.

NOTE: To roast lamb, preheat oven to 325°F. Place lamb on rack in roasting pan. Roast about 1½ hours or to desired doneness. Cover loosely with foil; let rest 5 to 10 minutes.

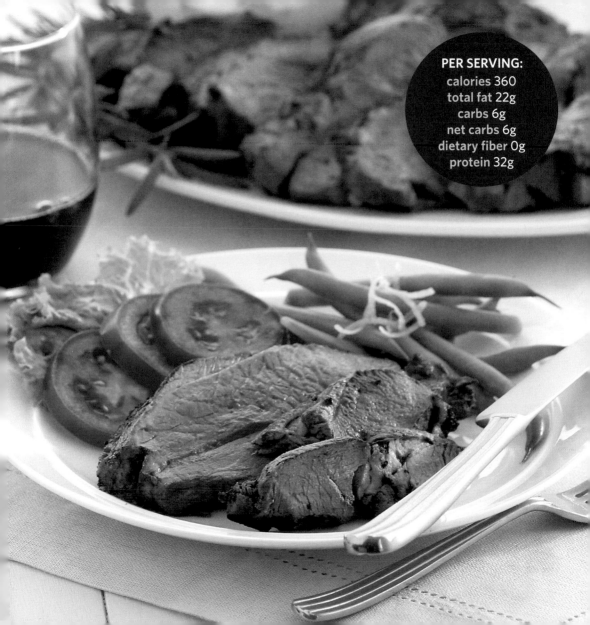

PER SERVING:
calories 360
total fat 22g
carbs 6g
net carbs 6g
dietary fiber 0g
protein 32g

Spicy Lemony Almond Chicken

MAKES 4 SERVINGS

½ teaspoon paprika

½ teaspoon black pepper

¼ teaspoon salt

4 boneless skinless chicken breasts (6 to 8 ounces each), flattened to ¼-inch thickness

1 ounce slivered almonds, toasted

¼ cup water

2 tablespoons lemon juice

2 tablespoons butter

2 teaspoons Worcestershire sauce

½ teaspoon grated lemon peel

1. Combine paprika, pepper and salt in small bowl; sprinkle evenly over both sides of chicken.

2. Coat large nonstick skillet with nonstick cooking spray; heat over medium-high heat. Add chicken; cook 3 to 4 minutes per side or until no longer pink in center. Transfer to serving plate; sprinkle with almonds. Keep warm.

3. Add water, lemon juice, butter and Worcestershire sauce to skillet. Stir until pan sauces are reduced to ¼ cup, scraping bottom and side of skillet. Remove from heat; stir in lemon peel. Spoon evenly over chicken.

TIP: To pound chicken, place between 2 pieces of plastic wrap. Starting in the center, pound chicken with a meat mallet or rolling pin to reach an even thickness.

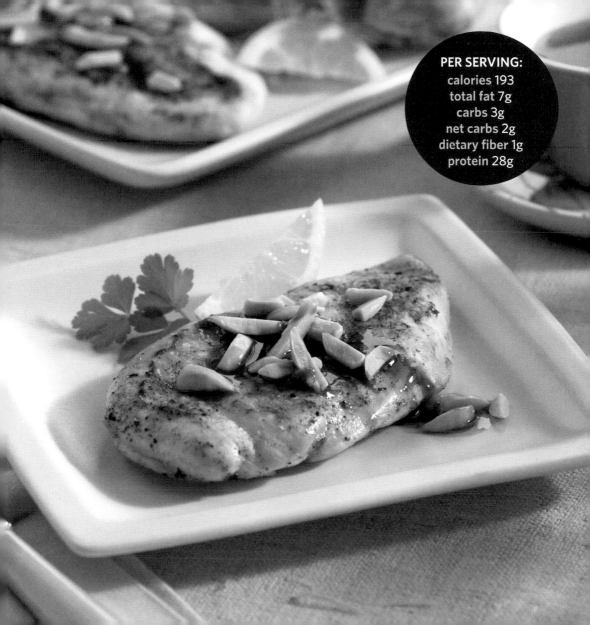

PER SERVING:
calories 193
total fat 7g
carbs 3g
net carbs 2g
dietary fiber 1g
protein 28g

Greek Chicken Burgers with Cucumber Yogurt Sauce

MAKES 4 SERVINGS

½ cup plus 2 tablespoons plain nonfat Greek yogurt

½ medium cucumber, peeled, seeded and finely chopped

Juice of ½ lemon

3 cloves garlic, minced, divided

2 teaspoons finely chopped fresh mint *or* ½ teaspoon dried mint

¼ teaspoon salt

⅛ teaspoon ground white pepper

1 pound ground chicken breast

3 ounces crumbled feta cheese

4 large kalamata olives, rinsed, patted dry and minced

1 egg

½ teaspoon dried oregano

¼ teaspoon black pepper

Mixed baby lettuce (optional)

1. Combine yogurt, cucumber, lemon juice, 2 cloves garlic, mint, salt and white pepper in medium bowl; mix well. Cover and refrigerate until ready to serve.

2. Combine chicken, cheese, olives, egg, oregano, black pepper and remaining 1 clove garlic in large bowl; mix well. Shape mixture into 4 patties.

3. Spray grill pan with nonstick cooking spray; heat over medium-high heat. Grill patties 5 to 7 minutes per side or until cooked through (165°F).

4. Serve burgers with sauce and mixed greens, if desired.

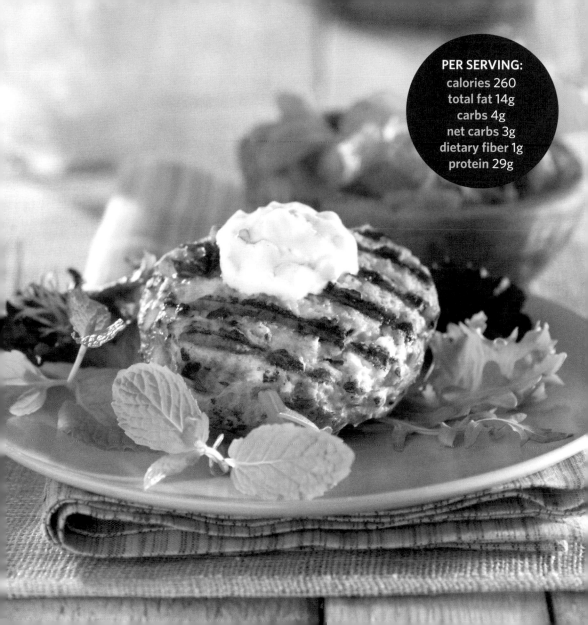

PER SERVING:
calories 260
total fat 14g
carbs 4g
net carbs 3g
dietary fiber 1g
protein 29g

Two-Cheese Sausage Pizza

MAKES 4 SERVINGS

1 pound sweet Italian turkey sausage

1 tablespoon olive oil

2 cups sliced mushrooms

1 small red onion, thinly sliced

1 small green bell pepper, cut into thin strips

¼ teaspoon salt

¼ teaspoon dried oregano

¼ teaspoon black pepper

½ cup pizza sauce

2 tablespoons tomato paste

½ cup shredded Parmesan cheese

1 cup (4 ounces) shredded mozzarella cheese

8 pitted black olives

1. Preheat oven to 400°F. Remove sausage from casings. Pat into 9-inch glass pie plate. Bake 10 minutes or until sausage is firm. Remove from oven and carefully pour off fat.

2. Meanwhile, heat oil in large skillet over medium-high heat. Add mushrooms, onion, bell pepper, salt, oregano and black pepper; cook and stir 10 minutes or until vegetables are very tender.

3. Combine pizza sauce and tomato paste in small bowl; stir until well blended. Spread over sausage crust. Spoon half of vegetables over tomato sauce. Sprinkle with Parmesan and mozzarella cheeses. Top with remaining vegetables. Sprinkle with olives. Bake 8 to 10 minutes or until cheese melts. Cut into wedges to serve.

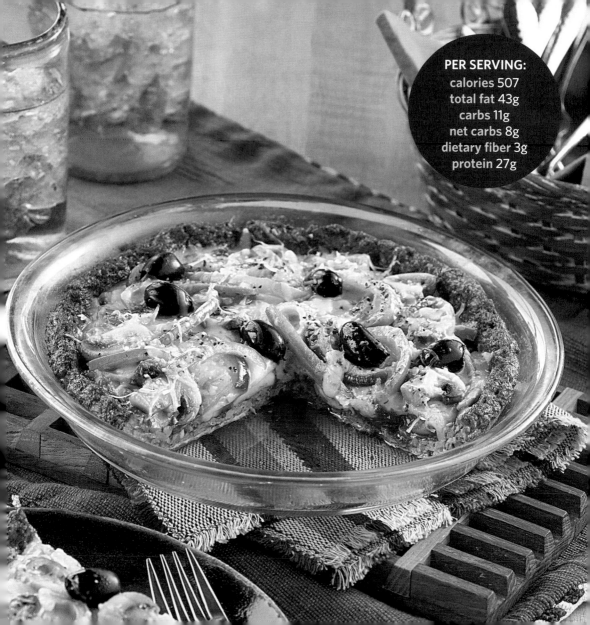

PER SERVING:
calories 507
total fat 43g
carbs 11g
net carbs 8g
dietary fiber 3g
protein 27g

Balsamic Chicken

MAKES 6 SERVINGS

1½ teaspoons fresh rosemary
    leaves, minced, *or*
    ½ teaspoon dried rosemary

 2 cloves garlic, minced

¾ teaspoon black pepper

½ teaspoon salt

 6 boneless skinless chicken
    breasts (6 to 8 ounces each)

 1 tablespoon olive oil

¼ cup balsamic vinegar

1. Combine rosemary, garlic, pepper and salt in small bowl; mix well. Place chicken in large bowl; drizzle chicken with oil and rub with spice mixture. Cover and refrigerate 2 to 3 hours.

2. Preheat oven to 450°F. Spray roasting pan or sheet pan with nonstick cooking spray. Place chicken in pan; bake 10 minutes. Turn chicken over, stirring in 3 to 4 tablespoons water if drippings begin to stick to pan. Bake about 10 minutes or until chicken is golden brown and no longer pink in center. If pan is dry, stir in another 1 to 2 tablespoons water to loosen drippings.

3. Drizzle vinegar over chicken in pan. Remove chicken to plates. Stir liquid in pan; drizzle over chicken.

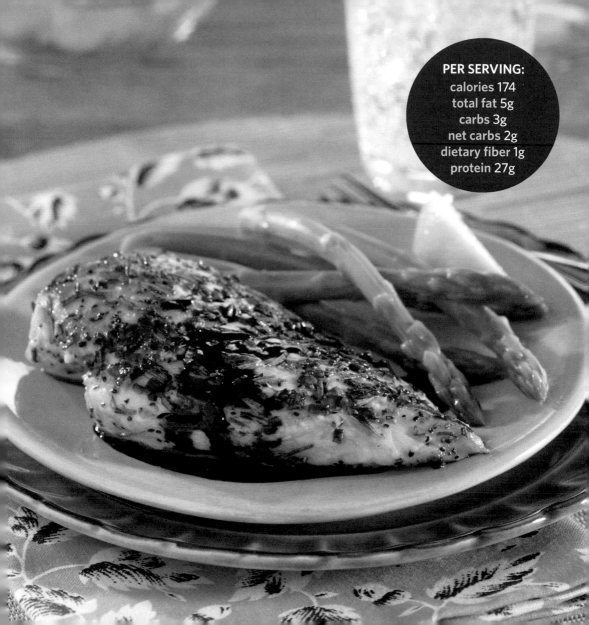

PER SERVING:
calories 174
total fat 5g
carbs 3g
net carbs 2g
dietary fiber 1g
protein 27g

Broiled Hunan Fish Fillets

MAKES 4 SERVINGS

3 tablespoons soy sauce
1 tablespoon finely chopped
    green onion
2 teaspoons dark sesame oil
1 clove garlic, minced

1 teaspoon minced fresh ginger
¼ teaspoon red pepper flakes
1 pound red snapper, scrod or
    cod fillets

1. Preheat broiler. Combine soy sauce, green onion, oil, garlic, ginger and red pepper flakes in small bowl.

2. Spray rack of broiler pan with nonstick cooking spray. Place fish on rack; brush with soy sauce mixture.

3. Broil 4 to 5 inches from heat 10 minutes or until fish begins to flake when tested with fork.

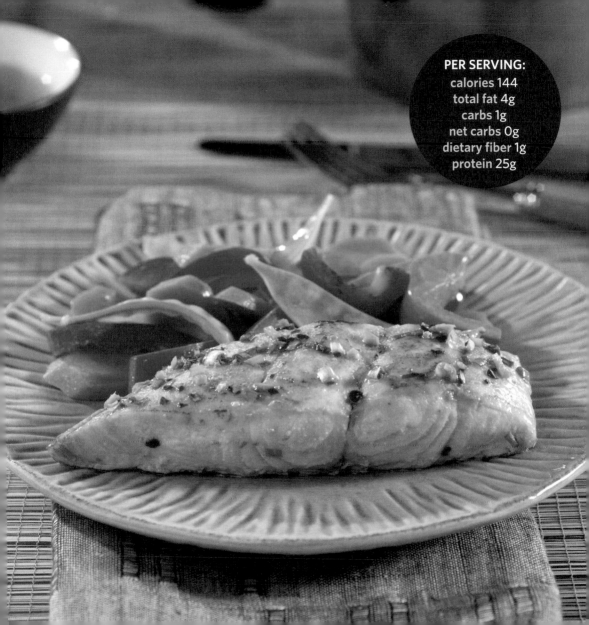

PER SERVING:
calories 144
total fat 4g
carbs 1g
net carbs 0g
dietary fiber 1g
protein 25g

Catfish with Bacon and Horseradish

MAKES 6 SERVINGS

6 **farm-raised catfish fillets (4 to 5 ounces each)**

2 **tablespoons butter**

¼ **cup chopped onion**

1 **package (8 ounces) cream cheese, softened**

¼ **cup dry white wine or vegetable broth**

2 **tablespoons prepared horseradish**

1 **tablespoon Dijon mustard**

½ **teaspoon salt**

⅛ **teaspoon black pepper**

4 **slices bacon, crisp-cooked and crumbled**

1. Preheat oven to 350°F. Grease large baking dish. Arrange fillets in single layer in prepared dish.

2. Melt butter in small skillet over medium-high heat. Add onion; cook and stir until softened. Combine cream cheese, wine, horseradish, mustard, salt and pepper in small bowl; stir in onion. Pour over fish and top with crumbled bacon.

3. Bake 30 minutes or until fish begins to flake when tested with fork. Serve immediately.

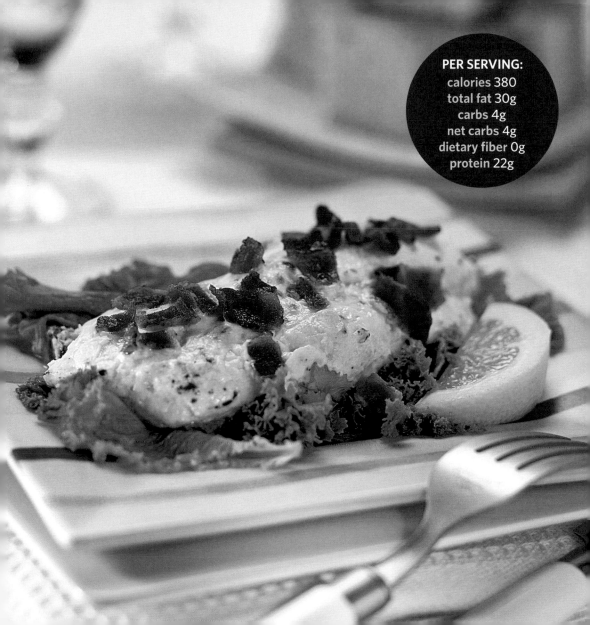

PER SERVING:
calories 380
total fat 30g
carbs 4g
net carbs 4g
dietary fiber 0g
protein 22g

Lemony Greek Chicken

MAKES 4 SERVINGS

1 whole chicken (about 3 to 4 pounds), cut up
1 tablespoon olive oil
2 teaspoons Greek seasoning

1 teaspoon salt
1 teaspoon black pepper
Juice of 1 lemon

1. Preheat oven to 400°F.

2. Brush chicken with oil; arrange in 2 large baking dishes, bone side down. Combine Greek seasoning, salt and pepper in small bowl; sprinkle half over chicken. Bake 30 minutes.

3. Turn chicken pieces over. Sprinkle with remaining seasoning mixture and lemon juice. Bake 30 minutes or until chicken is cooked through (165°F).

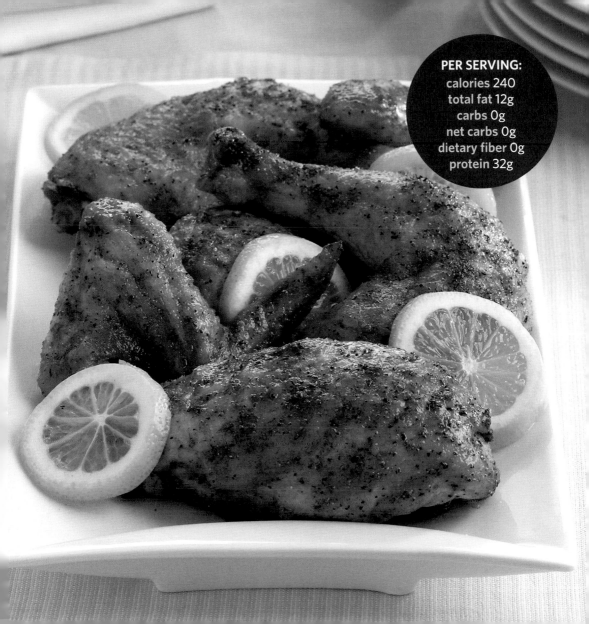

PER SERVING:
calories 240
total fat 12g
carbs 0g
net carbs 0g
dietary fiber 0g
protein 32g

Salmon with Bok Choy

MAKES 4 SERVINGS

4 skinless salmon fillets (4 ounces each)

3 tablespoons finely chopped fresh ginger

2 cloves garlic, minced

½ cup vegetable broth

3 tablespoons unseasoned rice vinegar

1 tablespoon soy sauce

6 cups chopped bok choy

1 teaspoon hoisin sauce

¼ cup sliced green onions

SLOW COOKER DIRECTIONS

1. Spray slow cooker with nonstick cooking spray. Arrange salmon in slow cooker; spread ginger and garlic evenly over salmon. Pour broth, vinegar and soy sauce over salmon. Cover; cook on LOW 1½ hours.

2. Add bok choy to slow cooker; cover and cook 30 minutes or until crisp-tender and salmon flakes easily when tested with fork.

3. Remove salmon from slow cooker; arrange on 4 plates. Stir hoisin sauce into liquid in slow cooker.

4. Spoon sauce evenly over salmon. Top with green onions. Serve with bok choy.

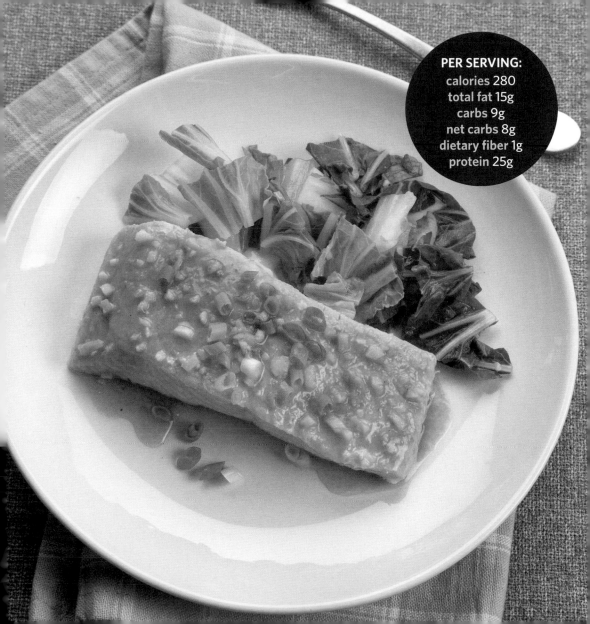

PER SERVING:
calories 280
total fat 15g
carbs 9g
net carbs 8g
dietary fiber 1g
protein 25g

Pork Medallions with Marsala

MAKES 4 SERVINGS

1 pound pork tenderloin, cut into
   ½-inch slices
   Salt and black pepper
2 tablespoons olive oil

1 clove garlic, minced
½ cup marsala wine
2 tablespoons chopped fresh
   parsley

1. Season pork with salt and pepper. Heat oil in large skillet over medium-high heat. Add pork; cook 3 minutes per side or until browned. Remove from skillet. Reduce heat to medium.

2. Add garlic to skillet; cook and stir 1 minute. Add wine and pork; cook 3 minutes or until pork is barely pink in center. Remove pork from skillet. Stir in parsley. Simmer wine mixture 2 to 3 minutes or until slightly thickened. Serve over pork.

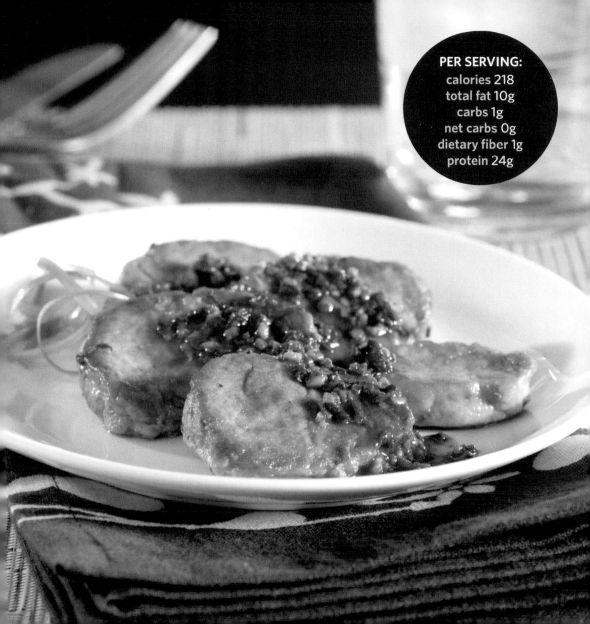

PER SERVING:
calories 218
total fat 10g
carbs 1g
net carbs 0g
dietary fiber 1g
protein 24g

Baked Fish with Thai Pesto

MAKES 6 SERVINGS

1 to 2 jalapeño peppers, coarsely chopped

1 lemon

1½ cups lightly packed fresh basil leaves

1 cup lightly packed fresh cilantro leaves

¼ cup lightly packed fresh mint leaves

¼ cup unsalted roasted peanuts

4 green onions, thinly sliced

3 cloves garlic, minced

2 tablespoons chopped fresh ginger

2 tablespoons unsweetened shredded coconut

½ cup peanut oil

2 pounds salmon fillets or other boneless fish fillets

1. Place jalapeño peppers in blender or food processor. Grate peel of lemon. Juice lemon to measure 2 tablespoons. Add peel and juice to blender.

2. Add basil, cilantro, mint, peanuts, green onions, garlic, ginger and coconut; blend until finely chopped. With motor running, slowly pour in oil; blend until mixed.

3. Preheat oven to 375°F. Rinse fish and pat dry with paper towels. Place fillets on lightly oiled baking sheet. Spread layer of pesto over each fillet.

4. Bake 10 minutes or until fish begins to flake when tested with fork and is just opaque in center.

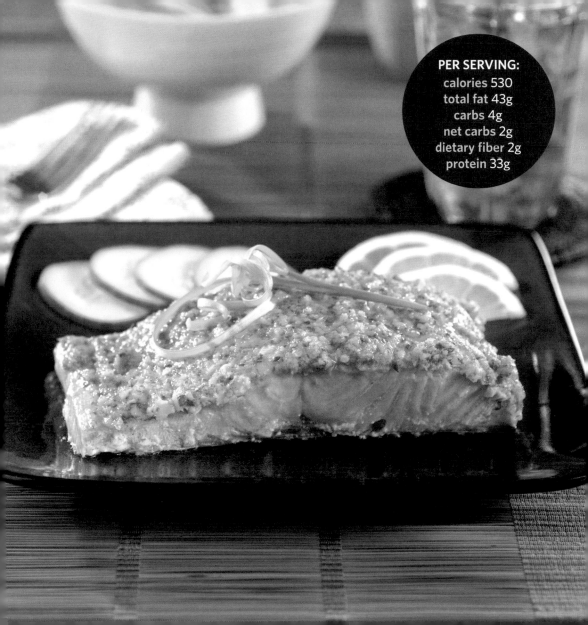

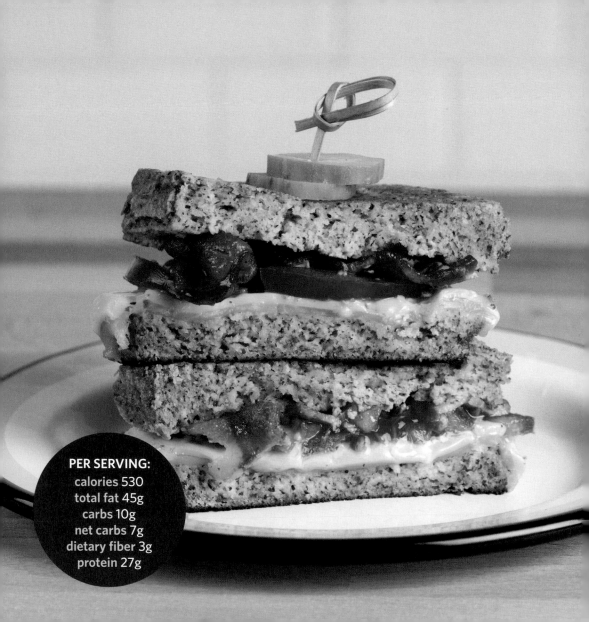

PER SERVING:
calories 530
total fat 45g
carbs 10g
net carbs 7g
dietary fiber 3g
protein 27g

Comfort Food

Bacon-Tomato Grilled Cheese

MAKES 4 SERVINGS

8 slices bacon, cut in half

4 slices sharp Cheddar cheese

4 slices Gouda cheese

8 tomato slices

½ loaf keto bread (page 138), cut into 8 slices

1 tablespoon butter

1. Cook bacon in large skillet over medium-high heat until crisp. Remove from skillet; drain on paper towels. Drain drippings from skillet; wipe out skillet with paper towels.

2. For each sandwich, layer 1 slice of Cheddar cheese, 1 slice of Gouda cheese, 2 tomato slices and 4 bacon slices between two bread slices. Melt 1 tablespoon butter in same skillet over medium heat. Add sandwiches; cook 3 to 4 minutes or until bottoms are toasted. Flip sandwiches. Reduce heat to medium-low; cover and cook 3 to 4 minutes or until bottoms are toasted and cheese is melted.

Noodle-Free Lasagna

MAKES 8 SERVINGS

1 medium eggplant

2 medium zucchini

2 medium summer squash

1¼ pounds sweet Italian turkey sausage, casings removed

2 medium bell peppers, diced

2 cups mushrooms, thinly sliced

1 can (about 14 ounces) diced tomatoes

1 cup tomato sauce

½ cup chopped fresh basil

1 teaspoon dried oregano

½ teaspoon salt

¼ teaspoon black pepper

1 container (15 ounces) whole-milk ricotta cheese

2 cups (8 ounces) shredded mozzarella cheese

¼ cup grated Parmesan cheese

1. Preheat oven to 375°F. Cut eggplant, zucchini and yellow squash lengthwise into ⅛- inch slices. Place on baking sheets. Bake 10 minutes. Set aside to cool.

2. Heat large nonstick skillet over medium-high heat. Add sausage; cook 8 to 10 minutes or until cooked through, stirring to break up meat. Drain fat. Transfer to plate. Add bell peppers and mushrooms to skillet; cook and stir 3 to 4 minutes or until vegetables are tender. Return sausage to skillet. Add tomatoes, tomato sauce, basil, oregano, salt and black pepper; cook and stir 1 to 2 minutes or until heated through.

3. Spray 13×9-inch baking dish with nonstick cooking spray. Layer one third of eggplant, zucchini and yellow squash in prepared baking dish. Spread half of ricotta over vegetables. Top with one third of tomato sauce mixture. Sprinkle evenly with half of mozzarella cheese. Repeat layers once, ending with final layer of vegetables and tomato sauce mixture. Sprinkle with Parmesan cheese; cover with foil.

4. Bake 45 minutes. Remove foil; bake 10 to 15 minutes or until vegetables are tender. Let stand 10 minutes before cutting.

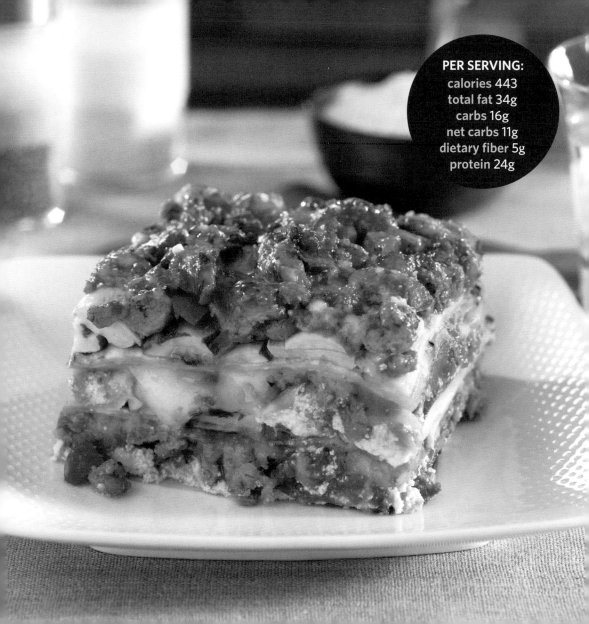

PER SERVING:
calories 443
total fat 34g
carbs 16g
net carbs 11g
dietary fiber 5g
protein 24g

Moussaka

MAKES 6 SERVINGS

1 eggplant (about 1 pound), cut into ¼-inch slices
2 tablespoons olive oil
1 pound ground beef
1 can (about 14 ounces) stewed tomatoes, drained
¼ cup red wine
2 tablespoons tomato paste
¾ teaspoon salt
½ teaspoon dried oregano
¼ teaspoon ground cinnamon, plus additional for garnish
¼ teaspoon black pepper
⅛ teaspoon ground allspice
½ (8-ounce) package cream cheese
¼ cup milk
¼ cup grated Parmesan cheese

1. Preheat broiler. Spray 8-inch square baking dish with nonstick cooking spray.

2. Line baking sheet with foil. Arrange eggplant slices on foil, overlapping slightly if necessary. Brush with oil; broil 5 to 6 inches from heat 4 minutes per side. *Reduce oven temperature to 350°F.*

3. Meanwhile, brown beef in large nonstick skillet over medium-high heat 6 to 8 minutes, stirring to break up meat. Drain fat. Add tomatoes, wine, tomato paste, salt, oregano, ¼ teaspoon cinnamon, pepper and allspice. Bring to a boil, breaking up large pieces of tomato with spoon. Reduce heat to medium-low; cover and simmer 10 minutes.

4. Place cream cheese and milk in small microwavable bowl. Cover and microwave on HIGH 1 minute. Stir until smooth.

5. Arrange half of eggplant slices in prepared baking dish. Spoon half of meat sauce over eggplant; sprinkle with half of Parmesan cheese. Repeat layers. Spoon cream cheese mixture evenly over top. Bake 20 minutes or until top begins to crack slightly. Sprinkle lightly with additional cinnamon, if desired. Let stand 10 minutes before serving.

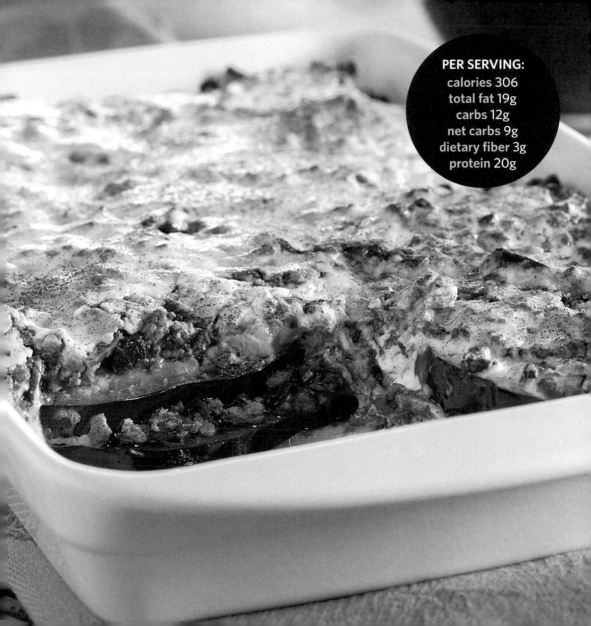

PER SERVING:
calories 306
total fat 19g
carbs 12g
net carbs 9g
dietary fiber 3g
protein 20g

Swiss Steak Stew

MAKES 10 SERVINGS

2 to 3 boneless beef top sirloin
   steaks (about 4 pounds)

2 cans (about 14 ounces each)
   diced tomatoes

2 green bell peppers, cut into
   ½-inch strips

2 medium onions, coarsely
   chopped

1 tablespoon seasoned salt

1 teaspoon black pepper

SLOW COOKER DIRECTIONS

Cut each steak into 3 to 4 pieces; place in slow cooker. Add tomatoes, bell peppers and onions. Sprinkle with seasoned salt and black pepper. Cover; cook on LOW 8 hours or until beef is tender.

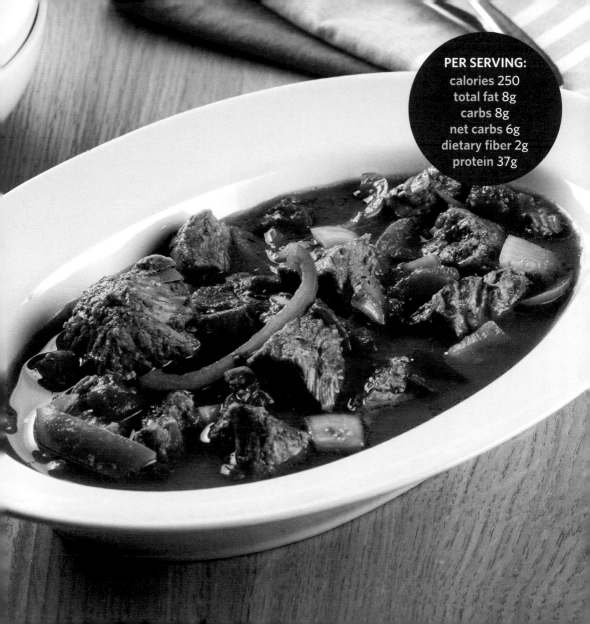

PER SERVING:
calories 250
total fat 8g
carbs 8g
net carbs 6g
dietary fiber 2g
protein 37g

Keto Bread

MAKES 1 LOAF (16 SLICES)

7 tablespoons butter, divided
2 cups almond flour
3½ teaspoons baking powder
½ teaspoon salt

6 eggs, at room temperature, separated*
¼ teaspoon cream of tartar

Discard 1 egg yolk.

1. Preheat oven to 375°F. Generously grease 8×4-inch loaf pan with 1 tablespoon butter. Melt remaining 6 tablespoons butter; cool slightly.

2. Combine almond flour, baking powder and salt in medium bowl. Add melted butter and 5 egg yolks; stir until blended.

3. Place egg whites and cream of tartar in bowl of stand mixer; attach whip attachment to mixer. Whip egg whites on high speed 1 to 2 minutes or until stiff peaks form.

4. Stir one third of egg whites into almond flour mixture until well blended. Gently fold in remaining egg whites until thoroughly blended. Scrape batter into prepared pan; smooth top.

5. Bake 25 to 30 minutes or until top is light brown and dry and toothpick inserted into center comes out clean. Cool in pan on wire rack 10 minutes. Remove from pan; cool completely.

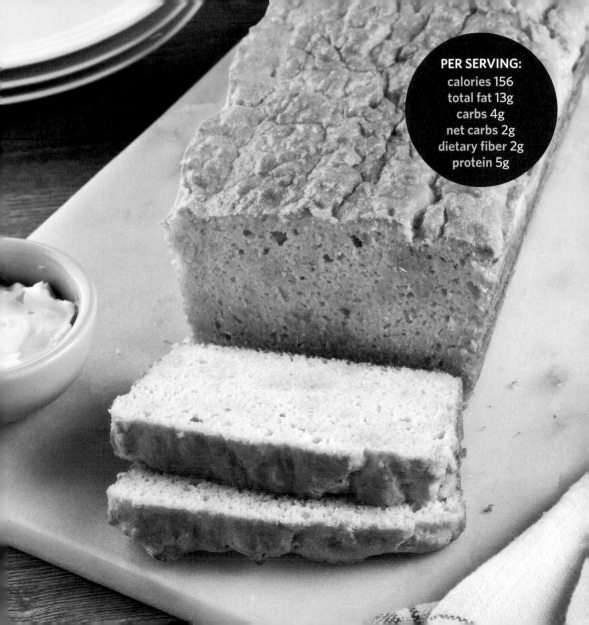

PER SERVING:
calories 156
total fat 13g
carbs 4g
net carbs 2g
dietary fiber 2g
protein 5g

Philly Cheese Steaks

MAKES 4 SERVINGS

2 tablespoons grapeseed oil, divided

1 green bell pepper, thinly sliced

1 medium onion, peeled and thinly sliced

½ teaspoon salt, divided

½ teaspoon black pepper, divided

¼ teaspoon red pepper flakes (optional)

1 pound boneless beef rib-eye steaks, sliced ¼ inch thick

4 slices American cheese

1. Heat 1 tablespoon oil in large nonstick skillet over high heat. Add bell pepper and onion; cook and stir 3 minutes or until tender. Sprinkle with ¼ teaspoon salt, ¼ teaspoon black pepper and red pepper flakes, if desired. Divide among 4 plates.

2. Heat remaining 1 tablespoon oil in same skillet. Sprinkle steaks with remaining ¼ teaspoon salt and ¼ teaspoon black pepper. Add steak to skillet; sprinkle with additional salt and black pepper, if desired. Cook and stir 3 minutes or until desired degree of doneness. Top with cheese; cook 1 minute or until cheese is melted. Place steak on vegetables.

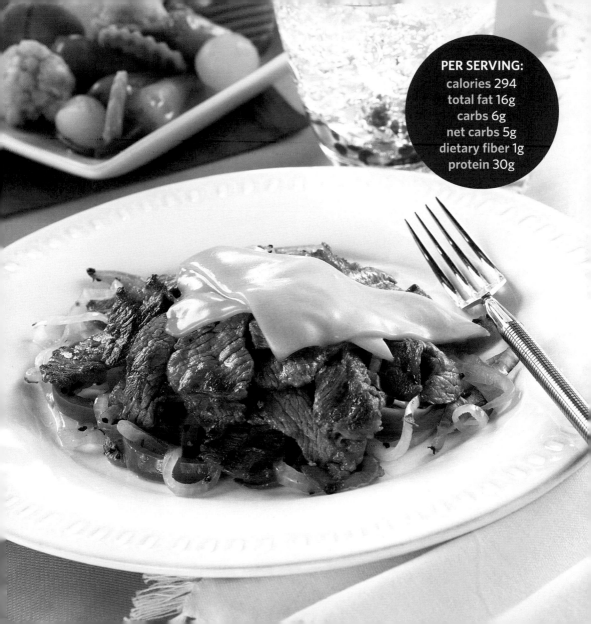

PER SERVING:
calories 294
total fat 16g
carbs 6g
net carbs 5g
dietary fiber 1g
protein 30g

Beefy Broccoli and Cheese Soup

MAKES 4 SERVINGS

4 ounces ground beef

2 cups beef broth

1 bag (10 ounces) frozen chopped broccoli, thawed

¼ cup chopped onion

1 cup whole milk

1 cup (4 ounces) shredded sharp Cheddar cheese

1½ teaspoons chopped fresh oregano *or* ½ teaspoon dried oregano

Salt and black pepper

Hot pepper sauce

1. Brown beef in large skillet over medium-high heat 6 to 8 minutes, stirring to break up meat. Drain fat.

2. Pour broth into medium saucepan; bring to a boil over medium-high heat. Add broccoli and onion; cook 5 minutes or until broccoli is tender. Stir milk and beef into saucepan; cook and stir until mixture is thickened and heated through.

3. Add cheese and oregano; stir until cheese is melted. Season with salt, black pepper and hot pepper sauce.

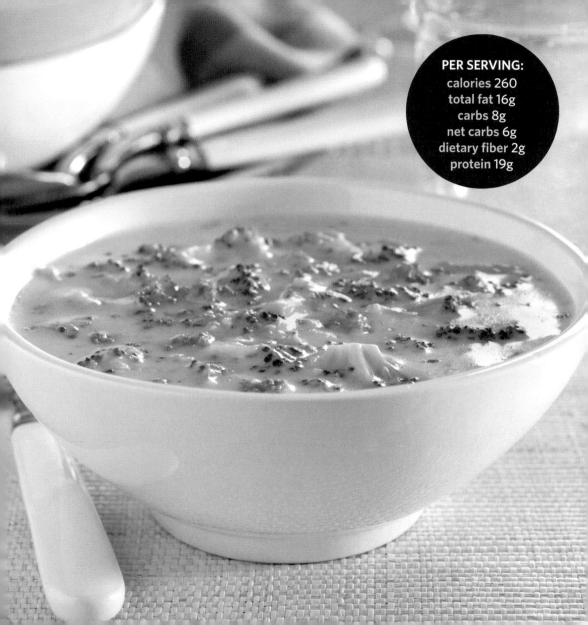

PER SERVING:
calories 260
total fat 16g
carbs 8g
net carbs 6g
dietary fiber 2g
protein 19g

Bacon Smashburger

MAKES 4 SERVINGS

4 slices bacon, cut in half
1 pound ground chuck
Salt and black pepper

4 slices sharp Cheddar cheese
4 eggs (optional)

1. Cook bacon in large skillet until crisp. Remove from skillet; drain on paper towels. Drain all but 1 tablespoon drippings from skillet.

2. Divide beef into 4 portions and shape lightly into loose balls. Place in same skillet over medium-high heat. Smash with spatula to flatten into thin patties; sprinkle with salt and pepper. Cook 2 to 3 minutes or until edges and bottoms are browned. Flip burgers and top with cheese. Cook 2 to 3 minutes for medium-rare or to desired degree of doneness. Transfer to plates.

3. If desired, crack eggs into hot skillet. Cook over medium heat about 3 minutes or until whites are opaque and yolks are desired degree of doneness, flipping once, if desired, for overeasy. Top burgers with eggs and bacon.

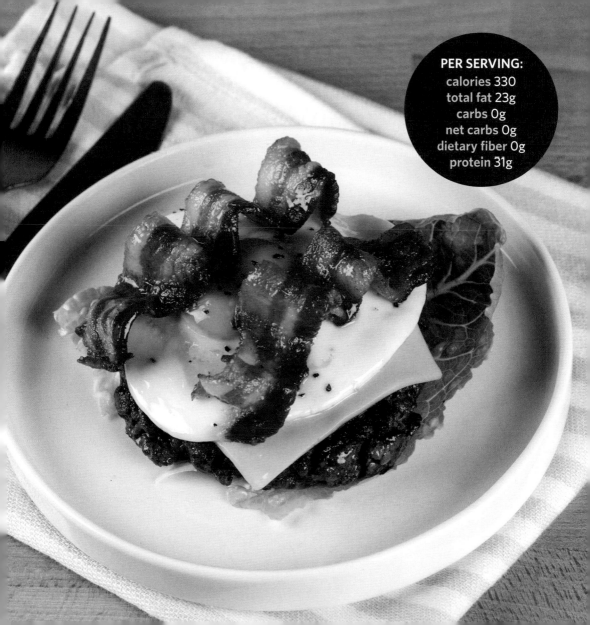

Pesto Turkey Meatballs

MAKES 4 SERVINGS

1 pound ground turkey

⅓ cup prepared pesto

⅓ cup grated Parmesan cheese, plus additional for garnish

¼ cup almond flour

1 egg

2 green onions, finely chopped

½ teaspoon salt, divided

2 tablespoons olive oil

2 cloves garlic, minced

⅛ teaspoon red pepper flakes

1 can (28 ounces) whole tomatoes, undrained, crushed with hands or coarsely chopped

1 tablespoon tomato paste

Cooked zucchini noodles (optional)

1. Combine turkey, pesto, ⅓ cup cheese, almond flour, egg, green onions and ¼ teaspoon salt in medium bowl; mix well. Shape mixture into 24 balls (about 1¼ inches). Refrigerate meatballs while preparing sauce.

2. Heat oil in large saucepan or Dutch oven over medium heat. Add garlic and red pepper flakes; cook and stir 2 minutes. Add tomatoes with liquid, tomato paste and remaining ¼ teaspoon salt; cook 5 minutes or until sauce begins to simmer, stirring occasionally.

3. Remove about 1 cup sauce from saucepan. Arrange meatballs in single layer in saucepan; pour reserved sauce over meatballs. Reduce heat to medium-low; cover and cook 20 minutes.

4. Uncover; increase heat to medium-high. Cook about 10 minutes or until sauce thickens slightly and meatballs are cooked through. Serve over zucchini noodles, if desired, and garnish with additional cheese.

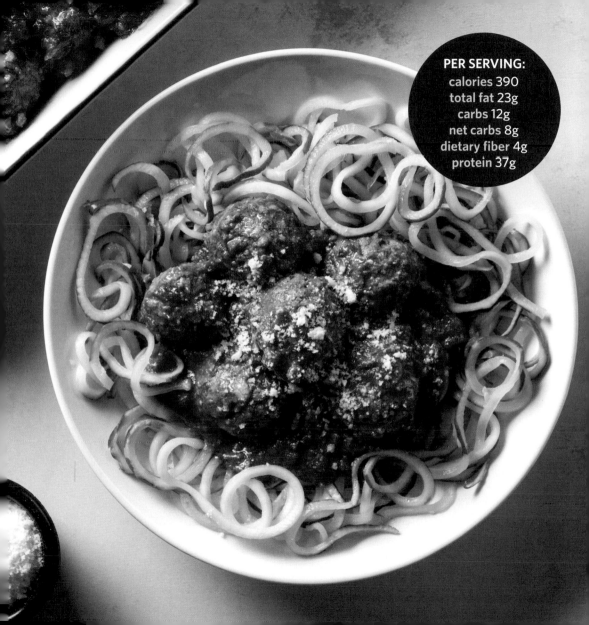

PER SERVING:
calories 390
total fat 23g
carbs 12g
net carbs 8g
dietary fiber 4g
protein 37g

Crab Dip

MAKES 3½ CUPS (¼ CUP PER SERVING)

½ **(8-ounce) package cream cheese, softened**

½ **cup sour cream**

2 **tablespoons mayonnaise**

¾ **teaspoon seasoned salt**

¼ **teaspoon paprika, plus additional for garnish**

2 **cans (6 ounces each) crabmeat, drained and flaked**

½ **cup (2 ounces) shredded mozzarella cheese**

2 **tablespoons minced onion**

2 **tablespoons finely chopped green bell pepper***

Chopped fresh parsley (optional)

*For a spicier dip, substitute 1 tablespoon minced jalapeño pepper for the bell pepper.

1. Preheat oven to 350°F.

2. Combine cream cheese, sour cream, mayonnaise, seasoned salt and ¼ teaspoon paprika in medium bowl; stir until well blended and smooth. Add crabmeat, mozzarella cheese, onion and bell pepper; stir until blended. Spread in small (1-quart) shallow baking dish.

3. Bake 15 to 20 minutes or until bubbly and top is beginning to brown. Garnish with additional paprika and parsley.

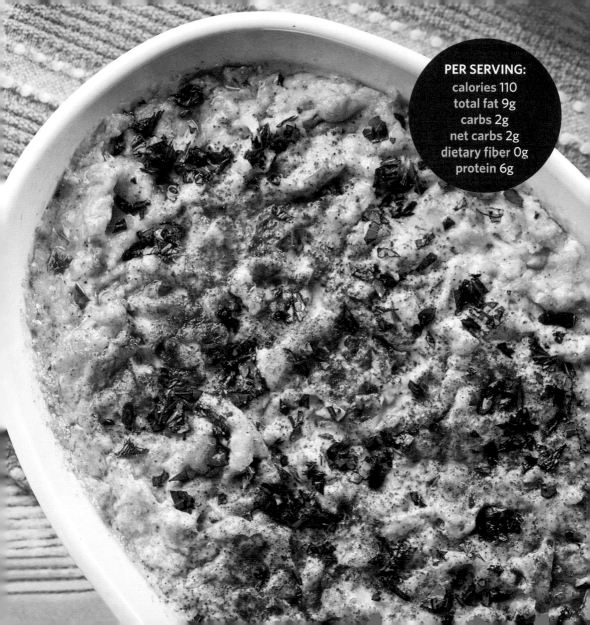

PER SERVING:
calories 110
total fat 9g
carbs 2g
net carbs 2g
dietary fiber 0g
protein 6g

Meatballs and Ricotta

MAKES 7 SERVINGS (21 MEATBALLS)

MEATBALLS

- 2 tablespoons olive oil
- ½ cup almond flour
- ½ cup milk
- 1 cup minced yellow onion
- 2 green onions, finely chopped
- ½ cup grated Romano cheese
- 2 eggs, beaten
- ¼ cup finely chopped fresh parsley
- ¼ cup finely chopped fresh basil
- 2 cloves garlic, minced
- 2 teaspoons salt
- ¼ teaspoon black pepper
- 1 pound ground beef
- 1 pound ground pork

SAUCE

- 2 tablespoons olive oil
- 2 tablespoons butter
- 1 cup finely chopped yellow onion
- 1 clove garlic, minced
- 1 can (28 ounces) whole Italian plum tomatoes, coarsely chopped, juice reserved
- 1 can (28 ounces) crushed tomatoes
- 1 teaspoon salt
- ¼ teaspoon black pepper
- ¼ cup finely chopped fresh basil
- 1 cup ricotta cheese

1. Preheat oven to 375°F. Brush 2 tablespoons oil over large rimmed baking sheet.

2. Combine almond flour and milk in large bowl; mix well. Add minced yellow onion, green onions, Romano, eggs, parsley, ¼ cup basil, 2 cloves garlic, 2 teaspoons salt and ¼ teaspoon black pepper; mix well. Add beef and pork; mix gently but thoroughly until blended. Shape mixture by ¼ cupfuls into balls (21 balls total). Place meatballs on prepared baking sheet; turn to coat with oil.

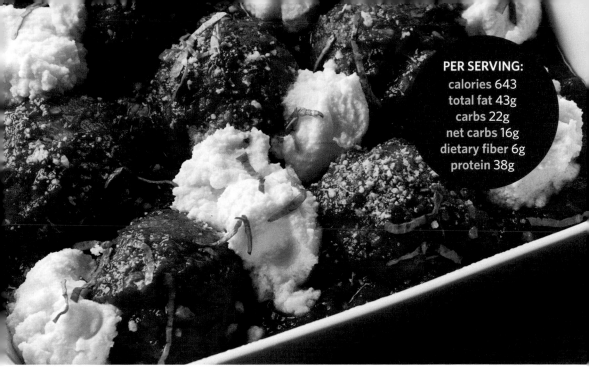

3. Bake about 20 minutes or until meatballs are cooked through (165°F). Meanwhile, prepare sauce.

4. Heat 2 tablespoons oil and butter in large saucepan over medium heat until butter is melted. Add 1 cup yellow onion; cook 8 minutes or until tender and lightly browned, stirring frequently. Add 1 clove garlic; cook and stir 1 minute or until fragrant. Add plum tomatoes with juice, crushed tomatoes, 1 teaspoon salt and ¼ teaspoon black pepper; bring to a simmer. Reduce heat to medium-low; cook 20 minutes, stirring occasionally.

5. Stir ¼ cup basil into sauce. Add meatballs; cook 10 minutes, stirring occasionally. Transfer meatballs and sauce to serving dish; dollop tablespoonfuls of ricotta between meatballs.

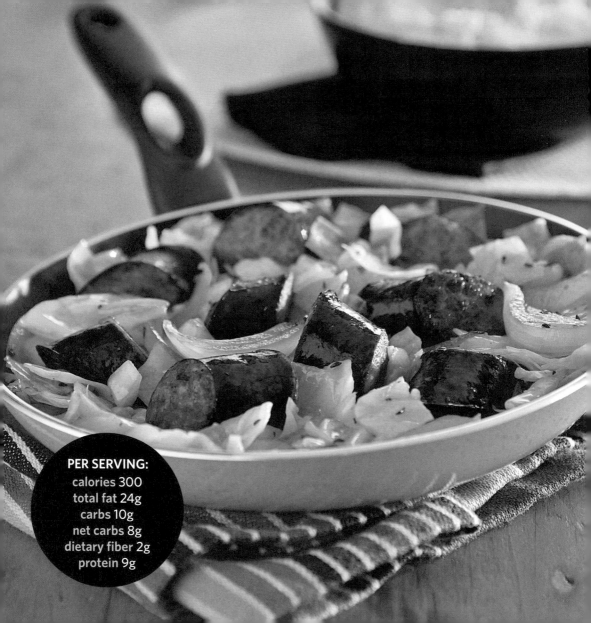

PER SERVING:
calories 300
total fat 24g
carbs 10g
net carbs 8g
dietary fiber 2g
protein 9g

Skillet and Sheet Pan Meals

Smoked Sausage and Cabbage

MAKES 6 SERVINGS

1 pound smoked sausage, cut into 2-inch pieces

1 tablespoon olive oil

6 cups coarsely chopped cabbage

1 yellow onion, cut into ½-inch wedges

2 cloves garlic, minced

¼ teaspoon caraway seeds

¼ teaspoon salt

¼ teaspoon black pepper

1. Cook and stir sausage in large nonstick skillet over medium-high heat 3 minutes or until browned. Transfer to plate.

2. Heat oil in same skillet. Add cabbage, onion, garlic, caraway seeds, salt and pepper; cook and stir 5 minutes or until onion begins to brown. Add sausage; cover and cook 5 minutes. Remove from heat; let stand 5 minutes.

Zesty Skillet Pork Chops

MAKES 4 SERVINGS

1 teaspoon chili powder

½ teaspoon salt, divided

4 boneless pork chops (about 1¼ pounds), well trimmed

2 cups diced tomatoes

1 cup chopped green, red or yellow bell pepper

¾ cup thinly sliced celery

½ cup chopped onion

1 tablespoon hot pepper sauce

1 teaspoon dried thyme

2 tablespoons finely chopped fresh parsley

1. Rub chili powder and ¼ teaspoon salt evenly over one side of pork chops.

2. Combine tomatoes, bell pepper, celery, onion, hot pepper sauce and thyme in medium bowl; mix well.

3. Spray large nonstick skillet with nonstick cooking spray; heat over medium-high heat. Add pork, seasoned side down; cook 1 minute. Turn pork. Top with tomato mixture; bring to a boil. Reduce heat to low. Cover; cook 25 minutes or until pork is tender and tomato mixture has thickened.

4. Transfer pork to serving plates. Bring tomato mixture to a boil over high heat; cook 2 minutes or until most liquid has evaporated. Remove from heat; stir in parsley and remaining ¼ teaspoon salt. Spoon sauce over pork.

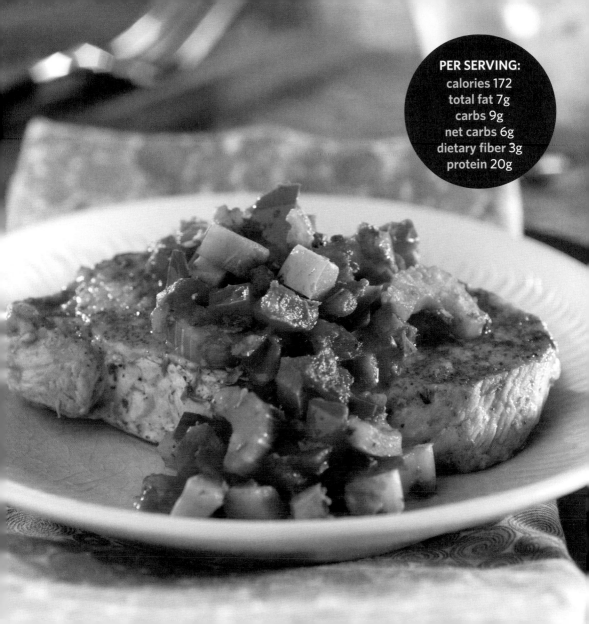

PER SERVING:
calories 172
total fat 7g
carbs 9g
net carbs 6g
dietary fiber 3g
protein 20g

Cheesy Chicken and Bacon

MAKES 4 SERVINGS

½ cup Dijon mustard

4 tablespoons olive oil, divided

1 teaspoon lemon juice

4 boneless skinless chicken breasts (6 to 8 ounces each)

Salt and black pepper

1 tablespoon butter

2 cups sliced mushrooms

4 slices bacon, cooked

½ cup (2 ounces) shredded Cheddar cheese

½ cup (2 ounces) shredded Monterey Jack cheese

Chopped fresh parsley

1. Whisk mustard, 3 tablespoons oil and lemon juice in medium bowl until well blended. Remove half of marinade mixture to use as sauce; cover and refrigerate until ready to serve.

2. Place chicken in large resealable food storage bag. Pour remaining half of marinade over chicken; seal bag and turn to coat. Refrigerate at least 2 hours.

3. Preheat oven to 375°F. Remove chicken from marinade; discard marinade. Heat remaining 1 tablespoon oil in large ovenproof skillet over medium-high heat. Add chicken; cook 3 to 4 minutes per side or until golden brown. (Chicken will not be cooked through.) Transfer chicken to plate; sprinkle with salt and pepper.

4. Heat butter in same skillet over medium-high heat. Add mushrooms; cook 8 minutes or until mushrooms begin to brown, stirring occasionally and scraping up browned bits from bottom of skillet. Season with salt and pepper. Return chicken to skillet; spoon mushrooms over chicken. Top with bacon; sprinkle with Cheddar and Monterey Jack.

5. Bake 8 to 10 minutes or until chicken is no longer pink in center and cheeses are melted. Sprinkle with parsley; serve with reserved mustard mixture.

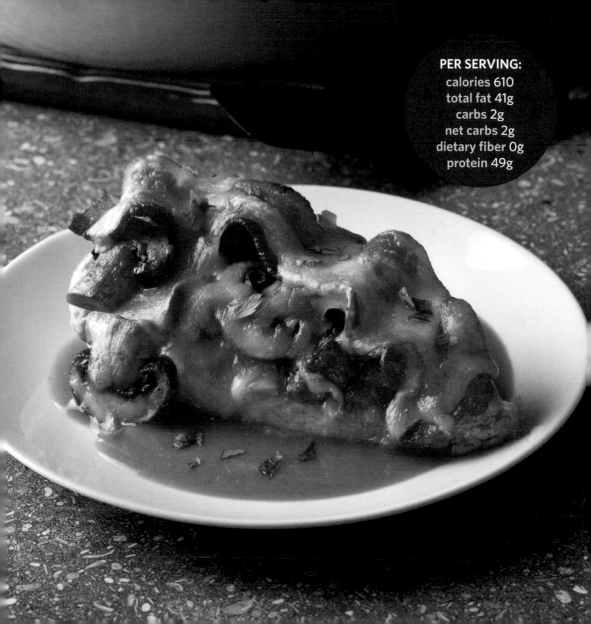

Pork Tenderloin with Cabbage and Leeks

MAKES 4 SERVINGS

- **1 teaspoon salt**
- **¾ teaspoon garlic powder**
- **½ teaspoon dried thyme**
- **½ teaspoon black pepper**
- **¼ cup olive oil**
- **1 pork tenderloin (about 1¼ pounds)**

- **½ medium savoy cabbage, cored and cut into ¼-inch slices (about 6 cups)**
- **1 small leek, cut in half lengthwise then cut crosswise into ¼-inch diagonal slices**
- **1 to 2 teaspoons cider vinegar**

1. Preheat oven to 450°F. Spray sheet pan with nonstick cooking spray.

2. Combine salt, garlic powder, thyme and pepper in small bowl; mix well. Stir in oil until well blended. Brush pork with about 1 tablespoon oil mixture, turning to coat all sides.

3. Combine cabbage and leek in large bowl. Drizzle with remaining oil mixture; toss to coat. Spread on prepared sheet pan; top with pork.

4. Roast about 25 minutes or until pork is 145°F, stirring cabbage mixture halfway through cooking time. Remove pork to cutting board; tent with foil and let stand 10 minutes before slicing. Add vinegar to cabbage mixture; stir to blend.

TIP: If you can't find savoy cabbage, you can substitute regular green cabbage but it may take slightly longer to cook. If the cabbage is not crisp-tender when the pork is done, return the vegetables to the oven for 10 minutes or until crisp-tender.

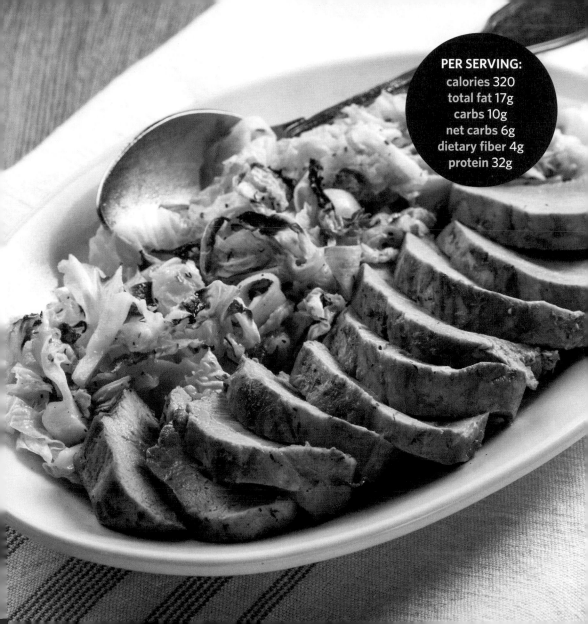

PER SERVING:
calories 320
total fat 17g
carbs 10g
net carbs 6g
dietary fiber 4g
protein 32g

Sausage and Peppers

MAKES 4 SERVINGS

1 pound uncooked hot or mild Italian sausage links

2 tablespoons olive oil

3 medium onions, cut into ½-inch slices

2 red bell peppers, cut into ½-inch slices

2 green bell peppers, cut into ½-inch slices

1½ teaspoons coarse salt, divided

1 teaspoon dried oregano

1. Fill medium saucepan half full with water; bring to a boil over high heat. Add sausage; cook 5 minutes over medium heat. Drain and cut diagonally into 1-inch slices.

2. Heat oil in large (12-inch) cast iron skillet over medium-high heat. Add sausage; cook about 10 minutes or until browned, stirring occasionally. Remove sausage to plate; set aside.

3. Add onions, bell peppers, 1 teaspoon salt and oregano to skillet; cook over medium heat about 25 minutes or until vegetables are very soft and browned in spots, stirring occasionally.

4. Stir sausage and remaining ½ teaspoon salt into skillet; cook 3 minutes or until heated through.

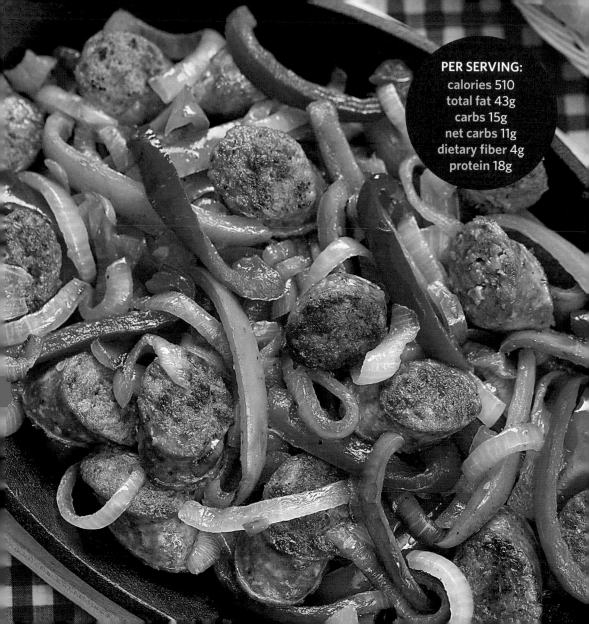

PER SERVING:
calories 510
total fat 43g
carbs 15g
net carbs 11g
dietary fiber 4g
protein 18g

Steak Fajitas

MAKES 4 SERVINGS

¼ cup lime juice

¼ cup soy sauce

4 tablespoons vegetable oil, divided

2 tablespoons Worcestershire sauce

2 cloves garlic, minced

½ teaspoon ground red pepper

1 pound flank steak, skirt steak or top sirloin

1 medium yellow onion, halved and cut into ¼-inch slices

1 green bell pepper, cut into ¼-inch strips

1 red bell pepper, cut into ¼-inch strips

Optional toppings: pico de gallo, guacamole, sour cream, shredded lettuce and shredded Cheddar cheese

1. Combine lime juice, soy sauce, 2 tablespoons oil, Worcestershire sauce, garlic and ground red pepper in medium bowl; mix well. Remove ¼ cup marinade to large bowl. Place steak in large resealable food storage bag. Pour remaining marinade over steak; seal bag and turn to coat. Marinate in refrigerator at least 2 hours or overnight. Add onion and bell peppers to bowl with ¼ cup marinade; toss to coat. Cover and refrigerate until ready to use.

2. Remove steak from marinade; discard marinade and wipe off excess from steak. Heat 1 tablespoon oil in large skillet (preferably cast iron) over medium-high heat. Cook steak about 4 minutes per side for medium rare or to desired doneness. Remove to cutting board; tent with foil and let rest 10 minutes.

3. Meanwhile, heat remaining 1 tablespoon oil in same skillet over medium-high heat. Add vegetable mixture; cook and stir about 8 minutes or until vegetables are crisp-tender and beginning to brown in spots. (Cook in 2 batches if necessary; do not pile vegetables in skillet.)

4. Thinly slice steak across the grain. Serve with vegetables, lime wedges and desired toppings.

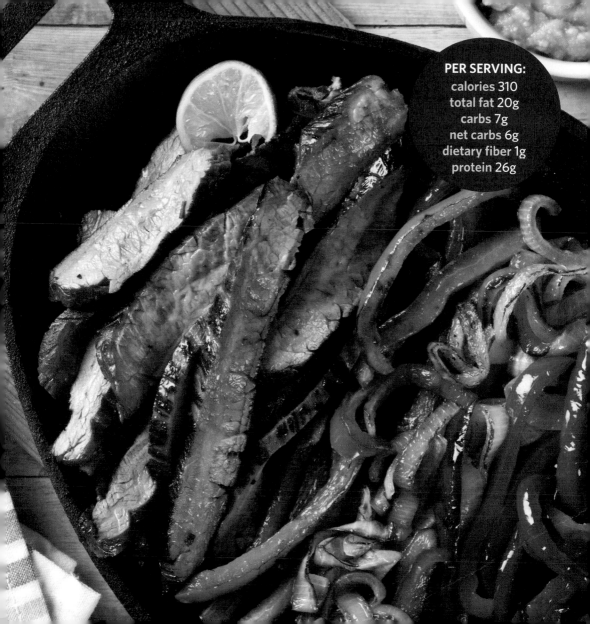

PER SERVING:
calories 310
total fat 20g
carbs 7g
net carbs 6g
dietary fiber 1g
protein 26g

Roasted Chicken
with Cabbage

MAKES 4 SERVINGS

⅓ cup olive oil

2 tablespoons red wine vinegar

2 cloves garlic, minced

1 teaspoon salt

1 teaspoon onion powder

¼ teaspoon paprika

¼ teaspoon black pepper

8 bone-in, skin-on chicken thighs (about 3 pounds)

1½ medium onions, cut into ½-inch slices (do not separate into rings)

1 small head green cabbage (about 1½ pounds)

Chopped fresh parsley

1. Preheat oven to 425°F. Spray sheet pan with nonstick cooking spray.

2. Whisk oil, vinegar, garlic, salt, onion powder, paprika and pepper in large bowl until well blended. Remove half of mixture to medium bowl; add chicken and turn to coat.

3. Add onion slices to large bowl with oil mixture; turn to coat. Arrange in single layer on prepared sheet pan. Cut cabbage in half through core (do not remove core). Cut each half into 1-inch wedges. Add cabbage to bowl with oil mixture; turn to coat. Arrange cabbage over onions on sheet pan.

4. Roast 50 to 55 minutes or until chicken is 165°F. Remove chicken to plate; tent with foil to keep warm. Carefully drain liquid from sheet pan. Stir vegetables; roast 10 to 15 minutes or until edges begin to brown and cabbage is crisp-tender. Serve chicken with vegetables. Garnish with parsley.

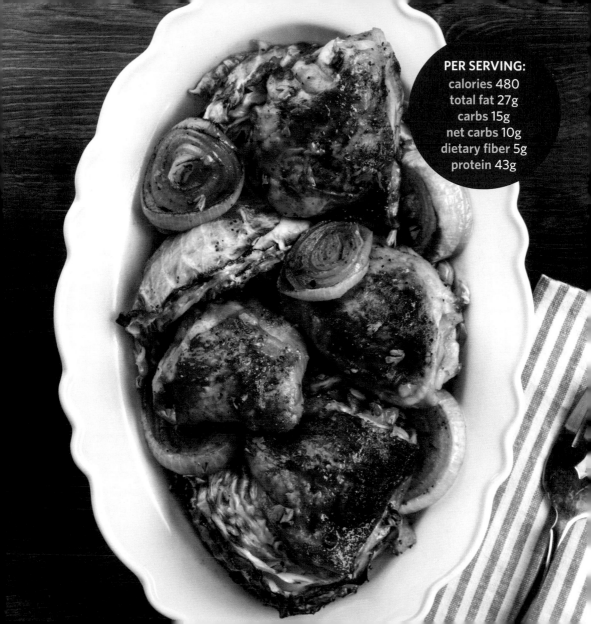

PER SERVING:
calories 480
total fat 27g
carbs 15g
net carbs 10g
dietary fiber 5g
protein 43g

Sheet Pan Chicken and Sausage Supper

MAKES 6 SERVINGS

⅓ cup olive oil

2 tablespoons balsamic vinegar

1 teaspoon salt

1 teaspoon garlic powder

½ teaspoon black pepper

¼ teaspoon red pepper flakes

3 pounds bone-in chicken thighs and drumsticks

1 pound sweet Italian sausage (4 to 5 links), cut diagonally into 2-inch pieces

6 small red onions (about 1 pound), each cut into 6 wedges

3½ cups broccoli florets

1. Preheat oven to 425°F. Line sheet pan with foil or spray with nonstick cooking spray.

2. Whisk oil, vinegar, salt, garlic powder, black pepper and red pepper flakes in small bowl until well blended. Combine chicken, sausage and onions on prepared sheet pan. Drizzle with oil mixture; toss until well coated. Spread meat and onions in single layer; turn chicken thighs skin side up.

3. Bake 30 minutes. Add broccoli to sheet pan; stir to coat broccoli with pan juices and turn sausage. Bake 30 minutes or until broccoli is beginning to brown and chicken is cooked through (165°F).

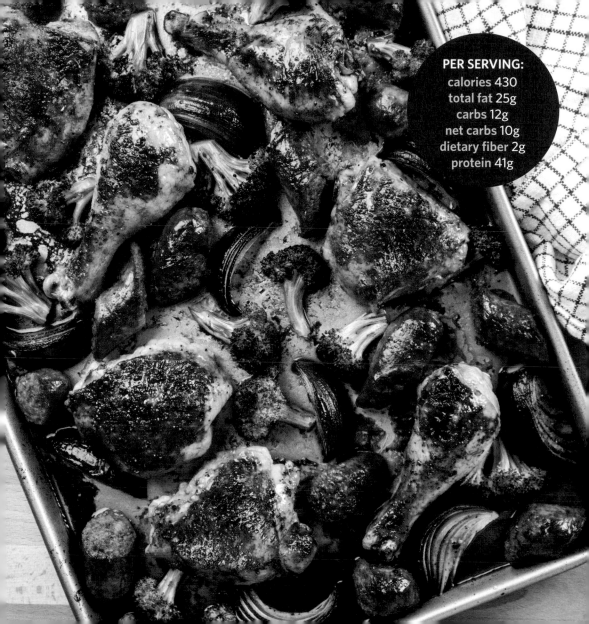

PER SERVING:
calories 430
total fat 25g
carbs 12g
net carbs 10g
dietary fiber 2g
protein 41g

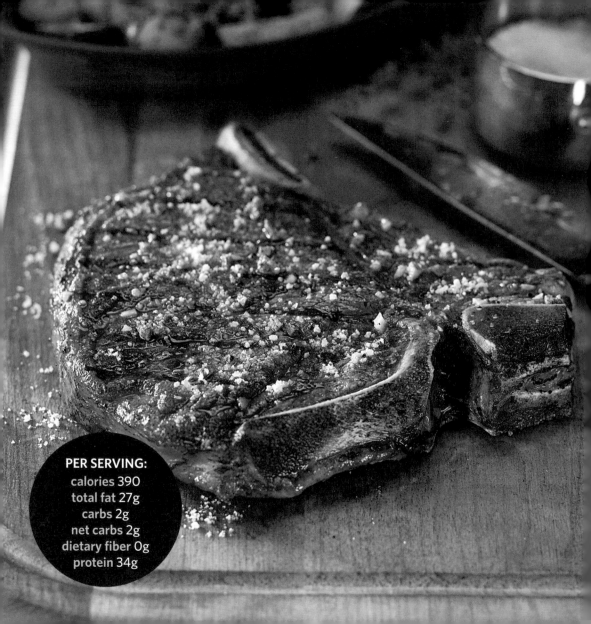

PER SERVING:
calories 390
total fat 27g
carbs 2g
net carbs 2g
dietary fiber 0g
protein 34g

Grill Recipes

Steak Parmesan

MAKES 2 SERVINGS

4 cloves garlic, minced
1 tablespoon olive oil
1 tablespoon coarse salt
1 teaspoon black pepper

2 beef T-bone or Porterhouse steaks, cut 1 to 1¼ inch thick (about 2 pounds)
¼ cup grated Parmesan cheese

1. Prepare grill for direct cooking. Combine garlic, oil, salt and pepper in small bowl; press into both sides of steaks. Let stand 15 minutes.

2. Place steaks on grid over medium-high heat. Grill, covered, 14 to 19 minutes or until internal temperature reaches 145°F for medium-rare doneness, turning once.

3. Transfer steaks to cutting board; sprinkle with cheese. Tent with foil; let stand 5 minutes. Serve immediately.

TIP: For a smoky flavor, soak 2 cups hickory or oak wood chips in cold water to cover at least 30 minutes. Drain and scatter over hot coals before grilling.

Szechuan Tuna Steaks

MAKES 4 SERVINGS

4 tuna steaks (6 ounces each),
    cut 1 inch thick

¼ cup dry sherry or sake

¼ cup soy sauce

1 tablespoon dark sesame oil

1 teaspoon hot chili oil *or*
    ¼ teaspoon red pepper
    flakes

1 clove garlic, minced

3 tablespoons chopped fresh
    cilantro (optional)

1. Place tuna in single layer in large shallow glass dish. Combine sherry, soy sauce, sesame oil, hot chili oil and garlic in small bowl. Reserve ¼ cup soy sauce mixture at room temperature. Pour remaining soy sauce mixture over fish; cover and marinate in refrigerator 40 minutes, turning once.

2. Spray grid with nonstick cooking spray. Prepare grill for direct cooking. Drain fish, discarding marinade.

3. Grill fish, uncovered, over medium-high heat 6 minutes or until tuna is seared but still feels somewhat soft in center,* turning halfway through grilling time. Remove to cutting board. Cut into thin slices; drizzle with reserved soy sauce mixture. Garnish with cilantro.

Tuna becomes dry and tough if overcooked. Cook to medium doneness for best results.

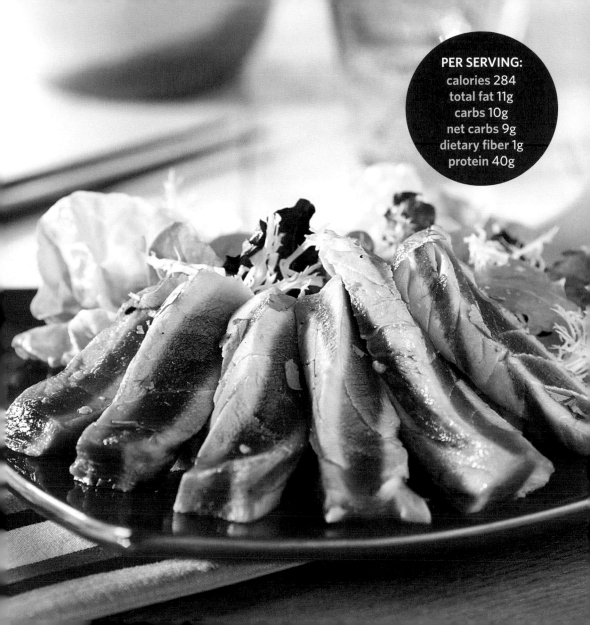

Fajita-Seasoned Grilled Chicken

MAKES 2 SERVINGS

2 boneless skinless chicken breasts (6 to 8 ounces each)
1 bunch green onions, ends trimmed

1 tablespoon olive oil
2 teaspoons fajita seasoning mix

1. Prepare grill for direct cooking.

2. Brush chicken and green onions with oil. Sprinkle both sides of chicken with seasoning mix. Grill chicken and green onions 6 to 8 minutes or until chicken is no longer pink in center. Serve chicken with green onions.

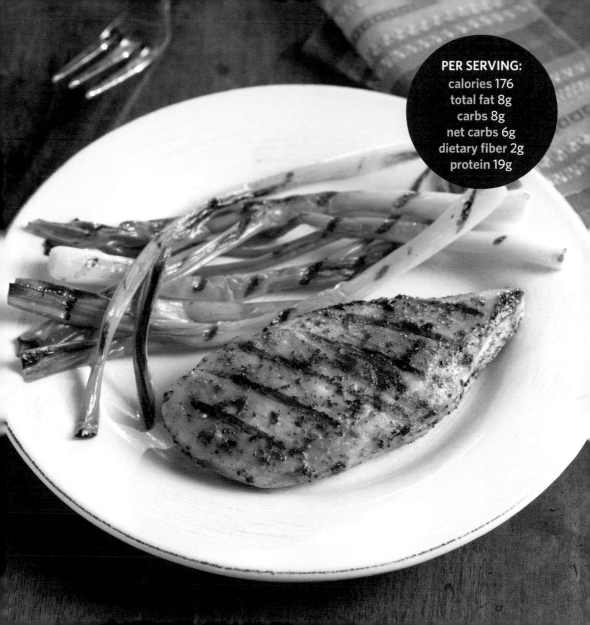

PER SERVING:
calories 176
total fat 8g
carbs 8g
net carbs 6g
dietary fiber 2g
protein 19g

Grilled Red Snapper with Avocado Salsa

MAKES 4 SERVINGS

1 teaspoon ground coriander

1 teaspoon paprika

¾ teaspoon salt

⅛ to ¼ teaspoon ground red pepper

½ cup diced ripe avocado

½ cup diced ripe papaya (optional)*

2 tablespoons chopped fresh cilantro

1 tablespoon lime juice

1 tablespoon olive oil

4 skinless red snapper or halibut fillets (5 to 7 ounces each)

4 lime wedges

*Or substitute with an additional ½ cup avocado.

1. Oil grid. Prepare grill for direct cooking. Combine coriander, paprika, salt and red pepper in small bowl; mix well.

2. For salsa, combine avocado, papaya, if desired, cilantro, lime juice and ¼ teaspoon spice mixture in medium bowl; set aside.

3. Brush oil over fish; sprinkle with remaining spice mixture. Grill fish, covered, over medium-high heat 10 minutes or until fish begins to flake when tested with fork, turning once. Serve with salsa and lime wedges.

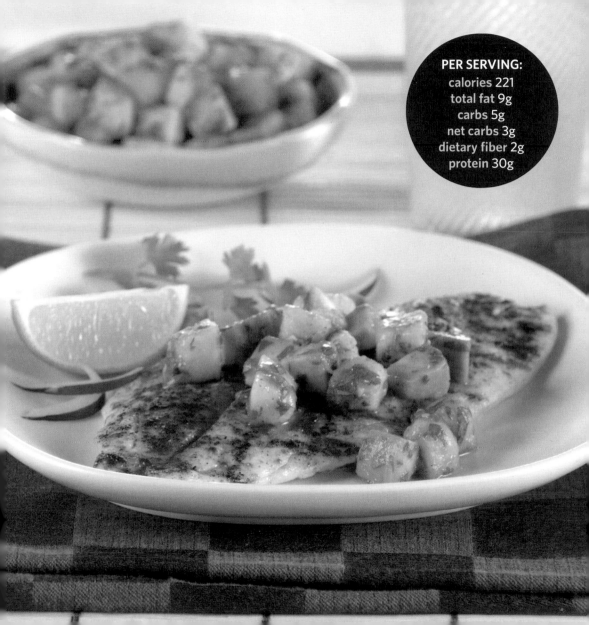

Moroccan-Style Lamb Chops

MAKES 4 SERVINGS

1 tablespoon olive oil
1 teaspoon ground cumin
1 teaspoon ground coriander
¾ teaspoon salt
⅛ teaspoon ground cinnamon

⅛ teaspoon ground red pepper
4 center-cut lamb loin chops, about 1 inch thick (1 pound total)
2 cloves garlic, minced

1. Prepare grill for direct cooking.

2. Combine oil, cumin, coriander, salt, cinnamon and red pepper in small bowl; mix well. Rub or brush oil mixture over both sides of lamb chops. Sprinkle garlic over both sides of lamb chops. Grill, covered, over medium-high heat 5 minutes per side for medium doneness.

HINT: This recipe also works well with an indoor, electric, countertop grill.

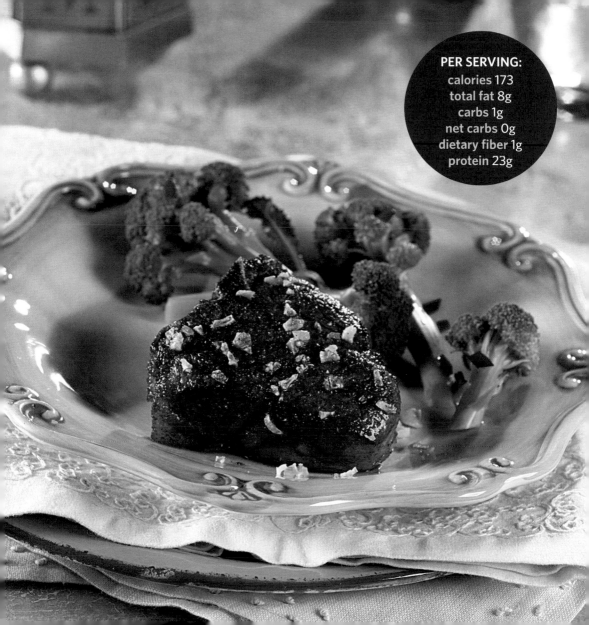

Grilled Strip Steaks
with Fresh Chimichurri

MAKES 4 SERVINGS

½ cup packed fresh basil leaves

⅓ cup extra virgin olive oil

¼ cup packed fresh parsley

2 tablespoons packed fresh cilantro

2 tablespoons fresh lemon juice

1 clove garlic

1¼ teaspoons salt, divided

½ teaspoon grated orange peel

¼ teaspoon ground coriander

¼ teaspoon plus ⅛ teaspoon black pepper, divided

4 bone-in strip steaks (8 ounces each), about 1 inch thick

¾ teaspoon ground cumin

1. For chimichurri, combine basil, oil, parsley, cilantro, lemon juice, garlic, ½ teaspoon salt, orange peel, coriander and ⅛ teaspoon pepper in food processor or blender; process until smooth.

2. Oil grid. Prepare grill for direct cooking. Sprinkle both sides of steaks with remaining ¾ teaspoon salt, cumin and remaining ¼ teaspoon pepper.

3. Grill steaks, covered, over medium-high heat 8 to 10 minutes for medium rare (145°F) or to desired doneness, turning once. Serve with chimichurri.

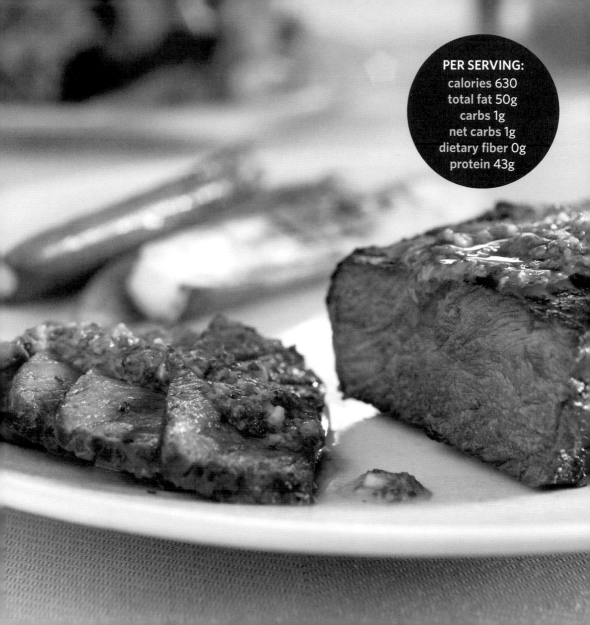

PER SERVING:
calories 630
total fat 50g
carbs 1g
net carbs 1g
dietary fiber 0g
protein 43g

Pesto-Stuffed Grilled Chicken

MAKES 6 SERVINGS

2 cloves garlic, peeled
½ cup packed fresh basil leaves
2 tablespoons pine nuts or walnuts, toasted*
¼ teaspoon black pepper
5 tablespoons extra virgin olive oil, divided

¼ cup grated Parmesan cheese
1 whole chicken (6 to 7 pounds)
2 tablespoons fresh lemon juice

*To toast pine nuts, spread in single layer in small heavy skillet. Cook and stir 2 to 3 minutes or until golden brown, stirring frequently.

1. Prepare grill with metal or foil drip pan. Bank briquettes on either side of drip pan for indirect cooking.

2. For pesto, drop garlic through feed tube of food processor with motor running. Add basil, pine nuts and black pepper; process until basil is minced. With motor running, add 3 tablespoons oil in thin steady stream until smooth paste forms, scraping down side of bowl once. Add cheese; process until well blended.

3. Remove giblets from chicken cavity. Loosen skin over breast of chicken by pushing fingers between skin and meat, taking care not to tear skin. Do not loosen skin over wings and drumsticks. Using rubber spatula or fingers, spread pesto under breast skin; massage skin to evenly spread pesto. Combine remaining 2 tablespoons oil and lemon juice in small bowl; brush over chicken. Tuck wings under back; tie legs together with kitchen string.

4. Place chicken, breast side up, on grid directly over drip pan. Grill, covered, over medium-low coals 1 hour 10 minutes to 1 hour 30 minutes or until thermometer inserted into thickest part of thigh not touching bone registers 185°F, adding 4 to 9 briquettes to both sides of the fire after 45 minutes to maintain medium-low coals. Transfer chicken to large cutting board; tent with foil. Let stand 15 minutes before carving.

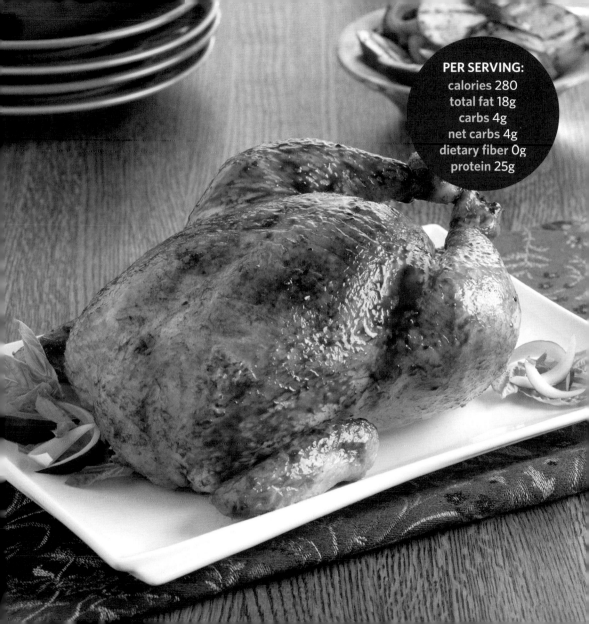

PER SERVING:
calories 280
total fat 18g
carbs 4g
net carbs 4g
dietary fiber 0g
protein 25g

Beef and Pepper Kabobs

MAKES 4 SERVINGS

8 ounces sirloin steak, trimmed of fat
1 clove garlic, minced
2 teaspoons soy sauce
2 teaspoons red wine vinegar
1½ teaspoons Dijon mustard

1 teaspoon olive oil
⅛ teaspoon black pepper
2 small bell peppers (green, red, yellow or orange)
4 large green onions, chopped
1 tablespoon chicken or vegetable broth

1. Slice steak into 16 (¼-inch) strips; place in glass bowl. Whisk garlic, soy sauce, vinegar, mustard, oil and black pepper in small bowl. Stir half of mixture into beef. Cover and refrigerate 2 to 3 hours, stirring occasionally. Cover and refrigerate remaining marinade.

2. Prepare grill for direct cooking. Core and seed bell peppers. Cut each into 12 chunks; thread onto 4 skewers. Grill 5 to 7 minutes per side or until well browned and tender. Grill green onions 3 to 5 minutes or until well browned on both sides. Stir broth into reserved marinade. Brush bell peppers and green onions lightly with marinade once during grilling.

3. Thread 4 beef strips onto 4 skewers. Grill 2 minutes per side, basting once per side with marinade. Place 1 beef skewer and 1 bell pepper skewer on each of 4 plates. Coarsely chop green onions and sprinkle over skewers.

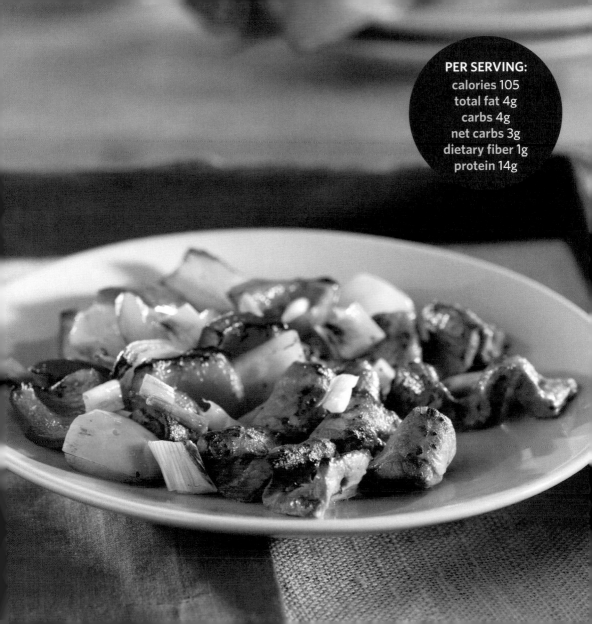

PER SERVING:
calories 105
total fat 4g
carbs 4g
net carbs 3g
dietary fiber 1g
protein 14g

Buffalo Chicken Drumsticks

8 large chicken drumsticks (about 2 pounds)

3 tablespoons hot pepper sauce

1 tablespoon vegetable oil

1 clove garlic, minced

¼ cup mayonnaise

3 tablespoons sour cream

1 tablespoon white wine vinegar

⅓ cup (about 1½ ounces) crumbled Roquefort or blue cheese

2 cups hickory chips

Celery sticks

1. Place chicken in large resealable food storage bag. Combine hot pepper sauce, oil and garlic in small bowl; pour over chicken. Seal bag; turn to coat. Marinate in refrigerator at least 1 hour or up to 24 hours for spicier flavor, turning occasionally.

2. For blue cheese dressing, combine mayonnaise, sour cream and vinegar in another small bowl. Stir in cheese; cover and refrigerate until serving.

3. Prepare grill for direct cooking. Meanwhile, soak hickory chips in cold water 20 minutes. Drain hickory chips; sprinkle over coals. Drain chicken; discard marinade.

4. Grill chicken, covered, over medium-high heat 25 to 30 minutes or until cooked through (165°F), turning occasionally. Serve with blue cheese dressing and celery sticks.

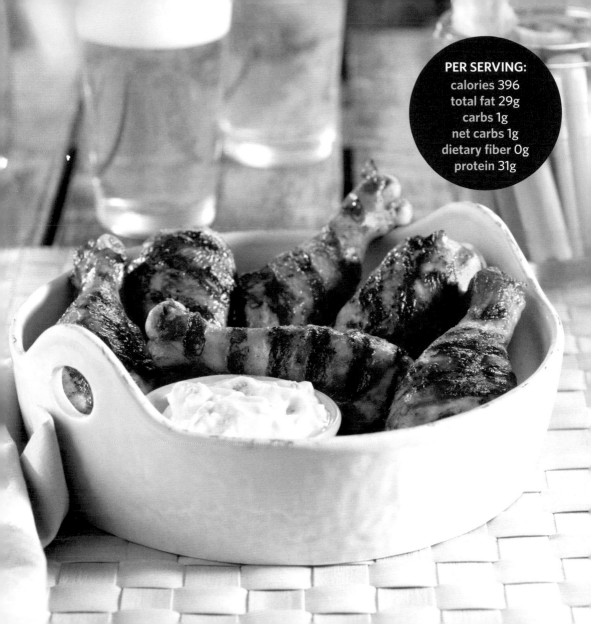

PER SERVING:
calories 396
total fat 29g
carbs 1g
net carbs 1g
dietary fiber 0g
protein 31g

Grilled Sesame Asparagus

MAKES 4 SERVINGS

1 **pound medium asparagus
    spears (about 20), trimmed**
1 **tablespoon sesame seeds**
2 **to 3 teaspoons balsamic
    vinegar**

¼ **teaspoon salt**
¼ **teaspoon black pepper**

1. Spray grid with nonstick cooking spray; prepare grill for direct cooking.

2. Place asparagus on baking sheet; spray lightly with cooking spray. Sprinkle with sesame seeds, rolling to coat.

3. Place asparagus on grid. Grill, uncovered, 4 to 6 minutes or until the asparagus begins to brown, turning once.

4. Transfer asparagus to serving dish. Sprinkle with vinegar, salt and pepper.

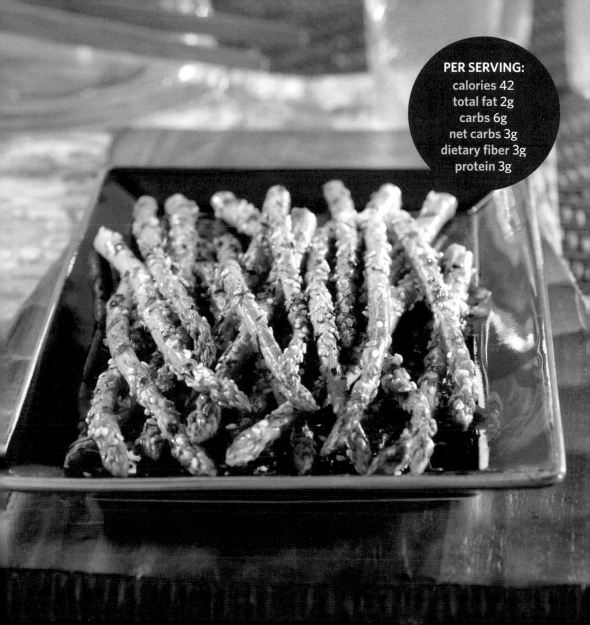

PER SERVING:
calories 42
total fat 2g
carbs 6g
net carbs 3g
dietary fiber 3g
protein 3g

Grilled Marinated Chicken

MAKES 8 SERVINGS

8 whole chicken legs, thighs and drumsticks attached (about 3½ pounds)

½ cup fresh lemon juice

¼ cup olive oil

2 tablespoons white wine vinegar

1 tablespoon grated lemon peel

2 cloves garlic, minced

1. Remove skin and all visible fat from chicken. Place chicken in 13×9-inch glass baking dish. Combine remaining ingredients in small bowl; blend well. Pour over chicken; turn to coat. Cover; refrigerate 3 hours or overnight, turning occasionally.

2. Spray grid with nonstick cooking spray. Prepare grill for direct cooking.

3. Grill chicken, covered, over medium-high heat 20 to 30 minutes or until cooked through (165°F), turning occasionally.

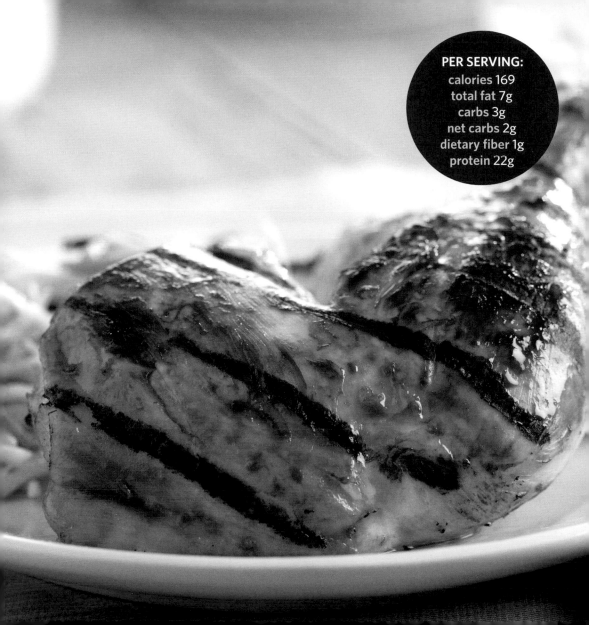

Lamb-Sicles

MAKES 4 SERVINGS

6 cloves garlic

1 teaspoon salt

2 tablespoons finely chopped fresh rosemary leaves

2 tablespoons olive oil

½ teaspoon ground black pepper

12 small lamb rib chops, bone-in and frenched*

*The term frenched means that the fat and meat have been cut away from the end of the bone protruding from the chop. Ask the butcher to do this for you if frenched chops are not available already cut. You can also purchase a frenched rack of lamb and cut it into individual chops.

1. Chop garlic with salt until finely minced. Place in small bowl; add rosemary, oil and pepper. Mix well.

2. Rub mixture over both sides of chops. Place on foil in single layer. Wrap and refrigerate 30 minutes to 3 hours.

3. Oil grid. Prepare grill for direct cooking. Grill chops over medium-high heat 2 to 5 minutes per side or until medium-rare (145°F). Lamb should feel slightly firm when pressed. (To check doneness, cut small slit in meat near bone; lamb should be rosy pink.)

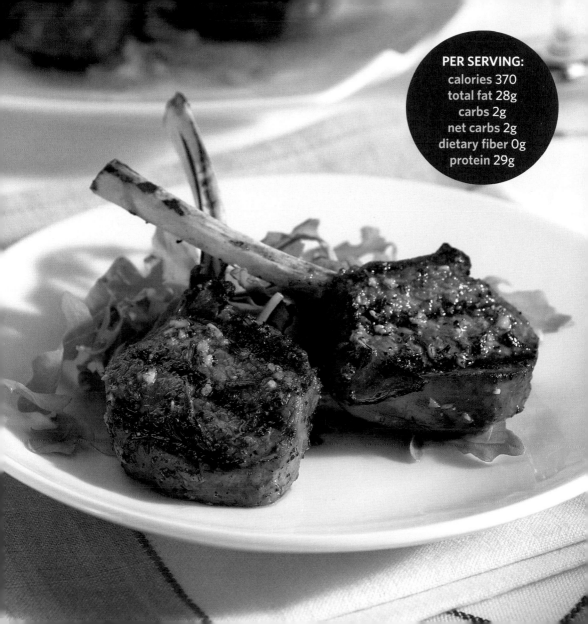

PER SERVING:
calories 370
total fat 28g
carbs 2g
net carbs 2g
dietary fiber 0g
protein 29g

Pollo Diavolo
(Deviled Chicken)

MAKES 4 SERVINGS

8 skinless bone-in chicken thighs
 (2½ to 3 pounds)
¼ cup olive oil
3 tablespoons lemon juice
6 cloves garlic, minced
1 to 2 teaspoons red pepper
 flakes

3 tablespoons butter, softened
1 teaspoon dried sage
1 teaspoon dried thyme
¾ teaspoon coarse salt
¼ teaspoon ground red pepper or
 black pepper
 Lemon wedges

1. Place chicken in large resealable food storage bag. Combine oil, lemon juice, garlic and red pepper flakes in small bowl. Pour mixture over chicken. Seal bag; turn to coat. Refrigerate at least 1 hour or up to 8 hours, turning once.

2. Prepare grill for direct cooking. Drain chicken; reserve marinade. Place chicken on grid; brush with reserved marinade. Grill, covered, over medium-high heat 8 minutes. Turn chicken; brush with remaining reserved marinade. Grill, covered, 8 to 10 minutes or until cooked through (165°F).

3. Meanwhile, combine butter, sage, thyme, salt and ground red pepper in small bowl; mix well. Transfer chicken to serving platter; spread herb butter over chicken. Serve with lemon wedges.

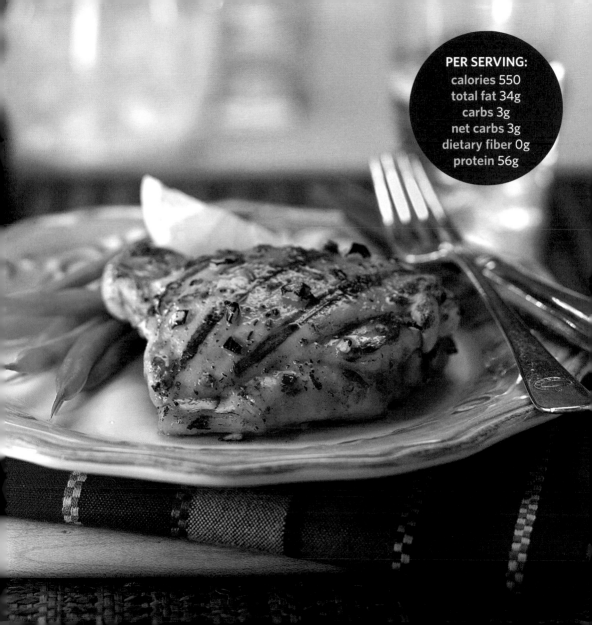

PER SERVING:
calories 550
total fat 34g
carbs 3g
net carbs 3g
dietary fiber 0g
protein 56g

Flank Steak
with Italian Salsa

MAKES 6 SERVINGS

- 2 tablespoons olive oil
- 2 teaspoons balsamic vinegar
- 1 flank steak (1½ pounds)
- 1 tablespoon minced garlic
- ¾ teaspoon salt, divided
- ¾ teaspoon black pepper, divided
- 1 cup diced plum tomatoes
- ⅓ cup chopped pitted kalamata olives
- 2 tablespoons chopped fresh basil

1. Whisk oil and vinegar in medium bowl until well blended. Place steak in shallow dish. Spread garlic over steak; sprinkle with ½ teaspoon salt and ½ teaspoon pepper. Spoon 2 tablespoons oil mixture over steak. Marinate in refrigerator at least 20 minutes or up to 2 hours.

2. Add tomatoes, olives, basil, remaining ¼ teaspoon salt and ¼ teaspoon pepper to remaining 2 teaspoons vinegar mixture in bowl; mix well.

3. Prepare grill for direct cooking. Remove steak from marinade, leaving garlic on steak. Discard marinade.

4. Grill steak over medium-high heat 5 to 6 minutes per side for medium-rare. Remove to cutting board; tent with foil and let stand 5 minutes. Cut steak diagonally across the grain into thin slices. Serve with tomato mixture.

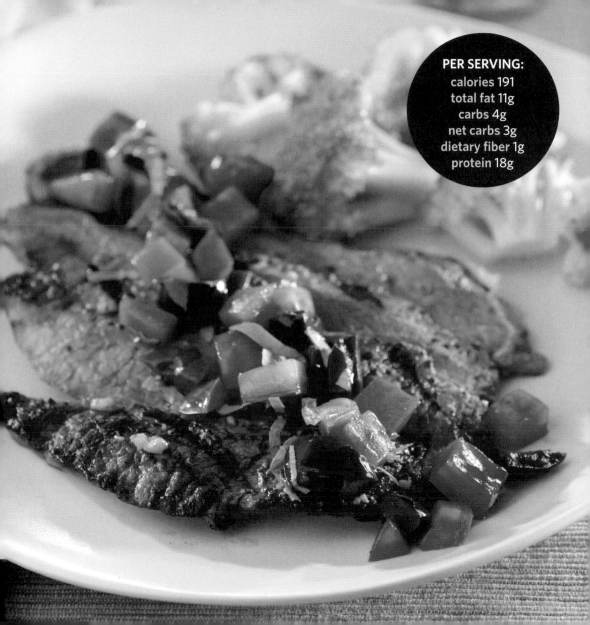

PER SERVING:
calories 191
total fat 11g
carbs 4g
net carbs 3g
dietary fiber 1g
protein 18g

Lobster Tails
with Tasty Butters

MAKES 4 SERVINGS

Hot & Spicy Butter, Scallion Butter or Chili-Mustard Butter (recipes follow)

4 fresh or thawed frozen lobster tails (about 5 ounces each)

1. Prepare grill for direct cooking. Prepare desired butters.

2. Rinse lobster tails in cold water. Butterfly tails by cutting lengthwise through centers of hard top shells and meat. Cut to, but not through, bottoms of shells. Press shell halves of tails apart with fingers. Brush lobster meat with butter mixture.

3. Place tails on grid, meat side down. Grill, uncovered, over medium-high heat 4 minutes. Turn tails meat side up. Brush with butter mixture; grill 4 to 5 minutes or until lobster meat turns opaque.

4. Heat remaining butter mixture, stirring occasionally. Serve butter mixture for dipping.

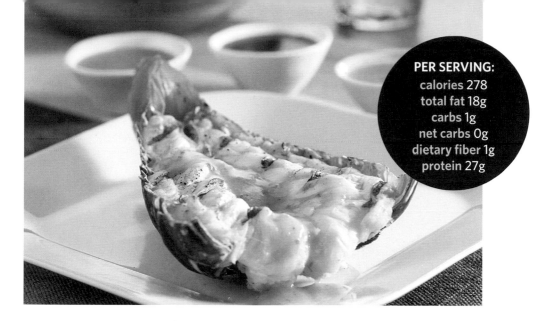

PER SERVING:
calories 278
total fat 18g
carbs 1g
net carbs 0g
dietary fiber 1g
protein 27g

Tasty Butters

HOT & SPICY BUTTER

- ⅓ cup butter, melted
- 1 tablespoon finely chopped onion
- 2 to 3 teaspoons hot pepper sauce
- 1 teaspoon dried thyme
- ¼ teaspoon ground allspice

SCALLION BUTTER

- ⅓ cup butter, melted
- 1 tablespoon finely chopped green onion top
- 1 tablespoon lemon juice
- 1 teaspoon freshly grated lemon peel
- ¼ teaspoon black pepper

CHILI-MUSTARD BUTTER

- ⅓ cup butter, melted
- 1 tablespoon finely chopped onion
- 1 tablespoon Dijon mustard
- 1 teaspoon chili powder

For each butter sauce, combine ingredients in small bowl.

Mustard-Grilled Red Snapper

MAKES 4 SERVINGS

½ **cup Dijon mustard**
1 **tablespoon red wine vinegar**
1 **teaspoon ground red pepper**

4 **red snapper fillets (about 6 ounces each)**

1. Spray grid with nonstick cooking spray. Prepare grill for direct cooking.

2. Combine mustard, vinegar and red pepper in small bowl; mix well. Coat fish thoroughly with mustard mixture.

3. Grill fish, covered, over medium-high heat 8 minutes or until fish begins to flake easily when tested with fork, turning halfway through grilling time.

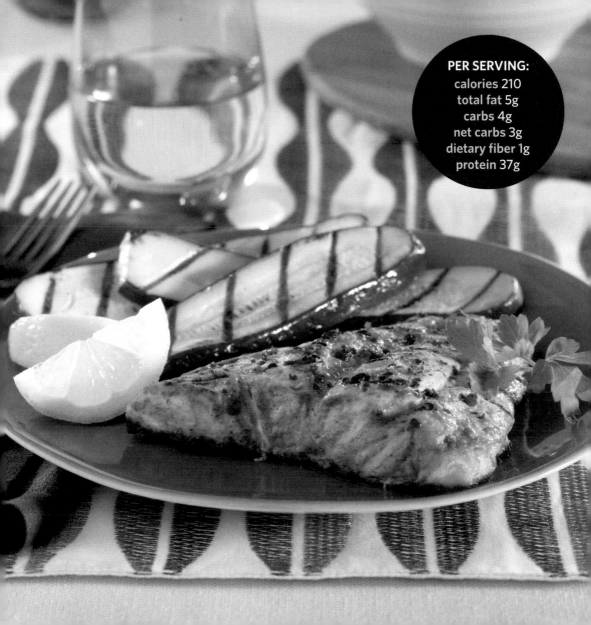

PER SERVING:
calories 210
total fat 5g
carbs 4g
net carbs 3g
dietary fiber 1g
protein 37g

Grilled Chicken Adobo

MAKES 4 SERVINGS

½ cup chopped onion

⅓ cup lime juice

6 cloves garlic

1 teaspoon ground cumin

1 teaspoon dried oregano

½ teaspoon dried thyme

¼ teaspoon ground red pepper

4 boneless skinless chicken breasts (6 to 8 ounces each)

3 tablespoons chopped fresh cilantro (optional)

1. Place onion, lime juice and garlic in food processor. Process until onion is finely minced. Transfer to large resealable food storage bag. Add cumin, oregano, thyme and ground red pepper; knead bag until blended. Place chicken in bag; press out air and seal. Turn to coat chicken with marinade. Refrigerate 30 minutes or up to 4 hours, turning occasionally.

2. Spray grid with nonstick cooking spray. Prepare grill for direct cooking. Remove chicken from marinade; discard marinade. Grill chicken 5 to 7 minutes per side over medium heat or until chicken is no longer pink in center. Transfer to clean serving platter and garnish with cilantro, if desired.

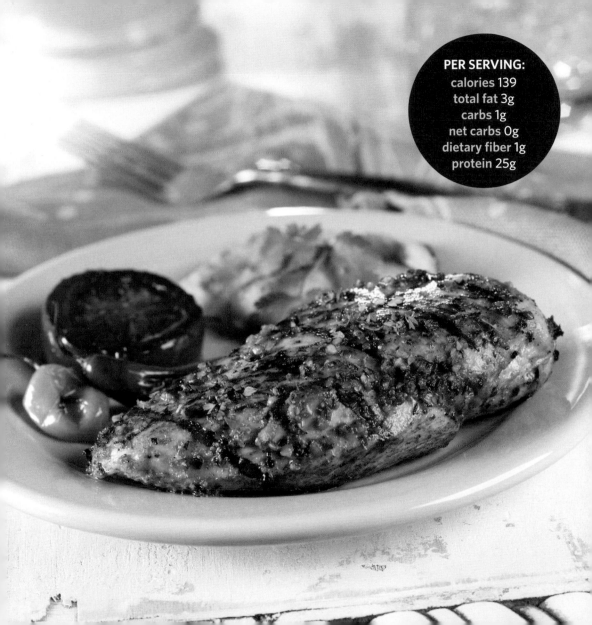

PER SERVING:
calories 139
total fat 3g
carbs 1g
net carbs 0g
dietary fiber 1g
protein 25g

Peppercorn Steaks

MAKES 4 SERVINGS

2 tablespoons olive oil

1 to 2 teaspoons cracked pink or black peppercorns or ground black pepper

1 teaspoon dried herbs, such as rosemary, oregano, basil or parsley

1 teaspoon minced garlic

4 boneless beef top loin (strip) or rib-eye steaks (6 ounces each)

¼ teaspoon salt

1. Combine oil, peppercorns, herbs and garlic in small bowl. Rub mixture on both sides of steaks. Place on plate; cover and refrigerate 30 to 60 minutes.

2. Prepare grill for direct cooking. Grill steaks, uncovered, over medium heat 10 to 12 minutes for medium-rare (145°F) to medium (160°F) or to desired doneness, turning once. Season with salt.

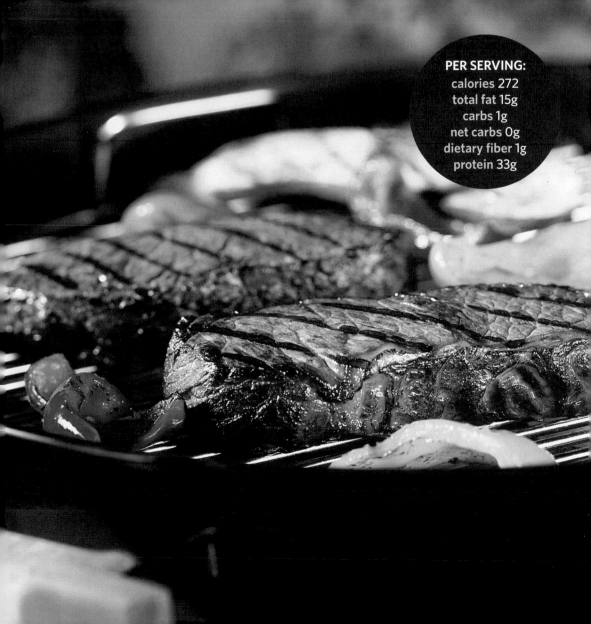

PER SERVING:
calories 272
total fat 15g
carbs 1g
net carbs 0g
dietary fiber 1g
protein 33g

Szechuan Grilled Mushrooms

MAKES 4 SERVINGS

1 pound large mushrooms
2 tablespoons soy sauce
2 teaspoons peanut oil
1 teaspoon dark sesame oil

1 clove garlic, minced
½ teaspoon crushed Szechuan peppercorns or red pepper flakes

1. Place mushrooms in large resealable food storage bag. Combine soy sauce, peanut oil, sesame oil, garlic and Szechuan peppercorns in small bowl; pour over mushrooms. Seal bag; turn to coat. Marinate at room temperature 15 minutes.

2. Prepare grill for direct cooking. Thread mushrooms onto skewers. Grill or broil mushrooms 5 inches from heat 10 minutes or until lightly browned, turning once. Serve immediately.

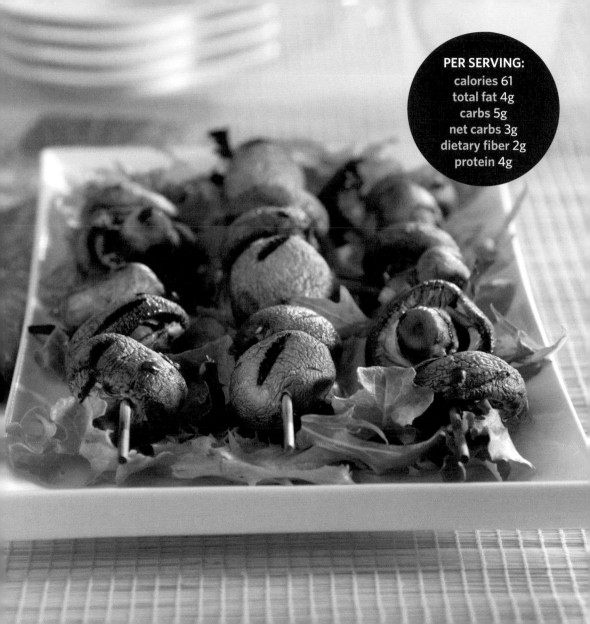

PER SERVING:
calories 61
total fat 4g
carbs 5g
net carbs 3g
dietary fiber 2g
protein 4g

Soy-Marinated Salmon

MAKES 4 SERVINGS

¼ **cup lime juice**

¼ **cup soy sauce**

1 **tablespoon grated fresh ginger**

1 **tablespoon minced garlic**

¼ **teaspoon black pepper**

4 **salmon fillets (7 to 8 ounces each)**

2 **tablespoons minced green onion**

1. Combine lime juice, soy sauce, ginger, garlic and pepper in medium bowl; mix well. Reserve ¼ cup mixture for serving; set aside. Place salmon in large resealable food storage bag. Pour remaining mixture over salmon; seal bag and turn to coat. Marinate in refrigerator 2 to 4 hours, turning occasionally.

2. Prepare grill for direct cooking. Remove salmon from marinade; discard marinade.

3. Grill salmon 10 minutes or until fish begins to flake when tested with fork. Brush with some of reserved marinade mixture; sprinkle with green onion.

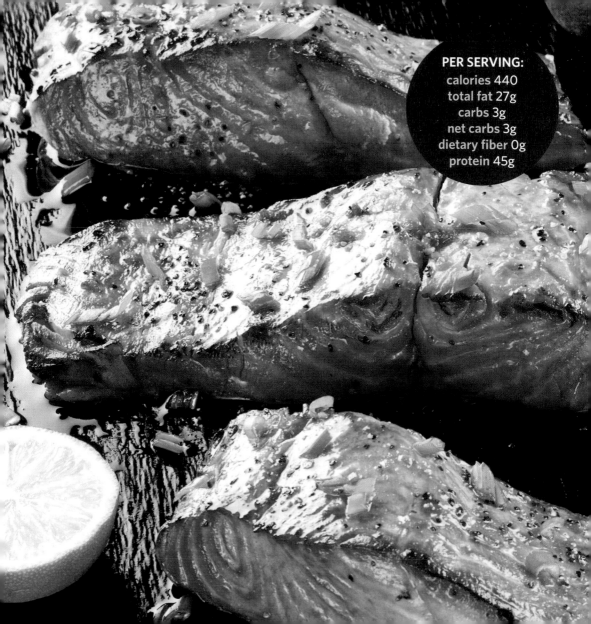

PER SERVING:
calories 440
total fat 27g
carbs 3g
net carbs 3g
dietary fiber 0g
protein 45g

Korean Beef Short Ribs

MAKES 6 SERVINGS

2½ pounds beef chuck flanken-style short ribs, cut ⅜ to ½ inch thick*

¼ cup chopped green onions

¼ cup water

¼ cup soy sauce

2 teaspoons grated fresh ginger

2 teaspoons dark sesame oil

2 cloves garlic, minced

½ teaspoon black pepper

1 tablespoon toasted sesame seeds

Flanken-style ribs can be ordered from your butcher. They are cross-cut short ribs sawed through the bones.

1. Place ribs in large resealable food storage bag. Combine green onions, water, soy sauce, ginger, oil, garlic and pepper in small bowl; pour over ribs. Seal bag; turn to coat. Marinate in refrigerator at least 4 hours or up to 8 hours, turning occasionally.

2. Prepare grill for direct cooking. Remove ribs from marinade; reserve marinade. Grill ribs, covered, over medium-high heat 5 minutes. Brush lightly with reserved marinade; turn and brush again. Discard remaining marinade. Continue to grill, covered, 5 to 6 minutes for medium (165°F) or to desired doneness. Sprinkle with sesame seeds.

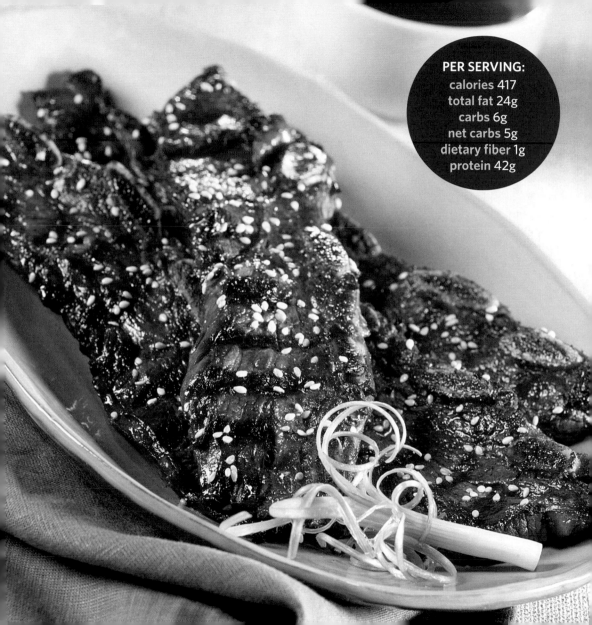

PER SERVING:
calories 417
total fat 24g
carbs 6g
net carbs 5g
dietary fiber 1g
protein 42g

French Quarter Steaks

MAKES 2 SERVINGS

½ cup water

2 tablespoons Worcestershire sauce

2 tablespoons soy sauce

1 tablespoon chili powder

3 cloves garlic, minced, divided

2 teaspoons paprika

1½ teaspoons ground red pepper

1¼ teaspoons black pepper, divided

1 teaspoon onion powder

2 top sirloin steaks (about 8 ounces each, 1 inch thick)

3 tablespoons butter, divided

1 tablespoon olive oil

1 large onion, thinly sliced

8 ounces sliced white or cremini mushrooms

¼ teaspoon plus ⅛ teaspoon salt, divided

1. Combine water, Worcestershire sauce, soy sauce, chili powder, 2 cloves garlic, paprika, red pepper, 1 teaspoon black pepper and onion powder in small bowl; mix well. Place steaks in large resealable food storage bag; pour marinade over steaks. Seal bag; turn to coat. Marinate in refrigerator 1 to 3 hours.

2. Remove steaks from marinade 30 minutes before cooking; discard marinade and pat steaks dry with paper towel. Oil grid. Prepare grill for direct cooking.

3. While grill is preheating, heat 1 tablespoon butter and oil in large skillet over medium high heat. Add onion; cook 5 minutes, stirring occasionally. Add mushrooms, ¼ teaspoon salt and remaining ¼ teaspoon black pepper; cook 10 minutes or until onion is golden brown and mushrooms are beginning to brown, stirring occasionally. Combine remaining 2 tablespoons butter, 1 clove garlic and ⅛ teaspoon salt in small skillet; cook over medium-low heat 3 minutes or until garlic begins to sizzle.

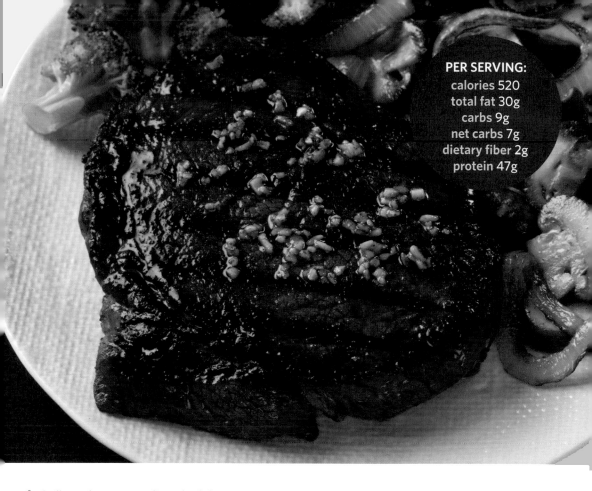

4. Grill steaks over medium-high heat 6 minutes; turn and grill 6 minutes for medium-rare or until desired doneness. Brush both sides of steaks with garlic butter during last 2 minutes of cooking. Remove to plate and tent with foil; let rest 5 minutes. Serve steaks with vegetable mixture.

Balsamic Grilled Pork Chops

MAKES 2 SERVINGS

2 tablespoons balsamic vinegar	⅛ teaspoon red pepper flakes
2 tablespoons soy sauce	2 boneless pork chops, trimmed of fat (8 ounces total)
1 teaspoon Dijon mustard	

1. Combine vinegar, soy sauce, mustard and red pepper flakes in small bowl. Stir until well blended. Reserve 1 tablespoon marinade; refrigerate until needed.

2. Place pork in large resealable food storage bag. Pour remaining marinade over pork. Seal bag; turn to coat. Refrigerate 2 hours or up to 24 hours.

3. Spray grill pan with nonstick cooking spray; heat over medium-high heat. Remove pork from marinade; discard marinade. Cook pork 4 minutes per side or until just slightly pink in center. Place on plates; top with reserved 1 tablespoon marinade.

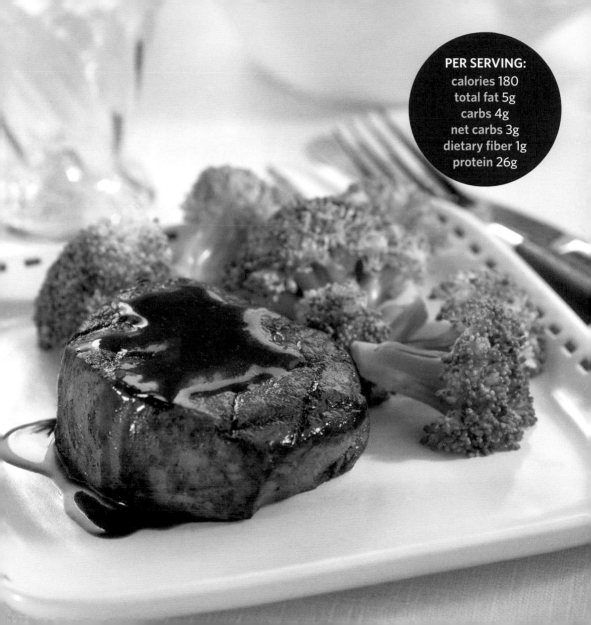

PER SERVING:
calories 180
total fat 5g
carbs 4g
net carbs 3g
dietary fiber 1g
protein 26g

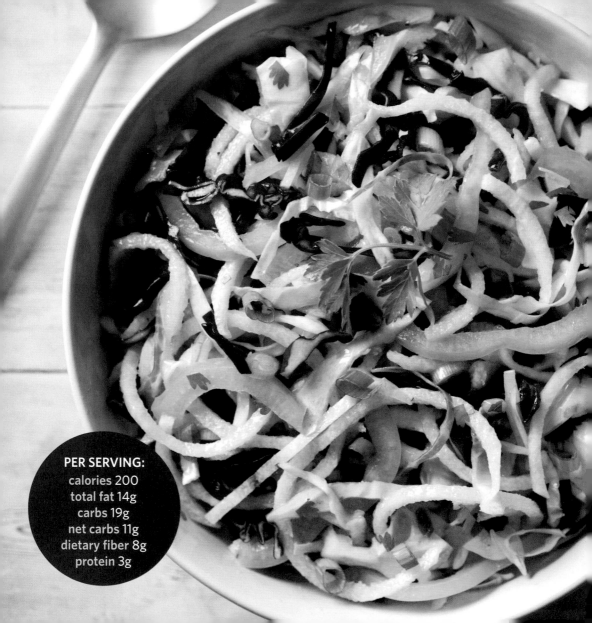

PER SERVING:
calories 200
total fat 14g
carbs 19g
net carbs 11g
dietary fiber 8g
protein 3g

Salads and Vegetables

Colorful Coleslaw

MAKES 8 SERVINGS

¼ head green cabbage, shredded or thinly sliced

¼ head red cabbage, shredded or thinly sliced

1 small yellow or orange bell pepper, thinly sliced

1 small jicama, peeled and julienned

¼ cup thinly sliced green onions

2 tablespoons chopped fresh cilantro

¼ cup vegetable oil

¼ cup fresh lime juice

1 teaspoon salt

⅛ teaspoon black pepper

1. Combine cabbage, bell pepper, jicama, green onions and cilantro in large bowl.

2. Whisk oil, lime juice, salt and black pepper in small bowl until well blended. Pour over vegetables; toss to coat. Cover and refrigerate 2 to 6 hours for flavors to blend.

Greek-Style Cucumber Salad

MAKES 4 SERVINGS

1 medium cucumber, peeled and diced
¼ cup chopped green onions
1 teaspoon minced fresh dill
1 small clove garlic, minced

1 cup sour cream
½ teaspoon salt
¼ teaspoon black pepper
⅛ teaspoon ground cumin
Lemon juice (optional)

1. Place cucumber, green onions, dill and garlic in salad bowl.

2. Combine sour cream, salt, pepper and cumin in small bowl; stir until blended. Stir sour cream mixture into cucumber mixture. Sprinkle with lemon juice to taste, if desired.

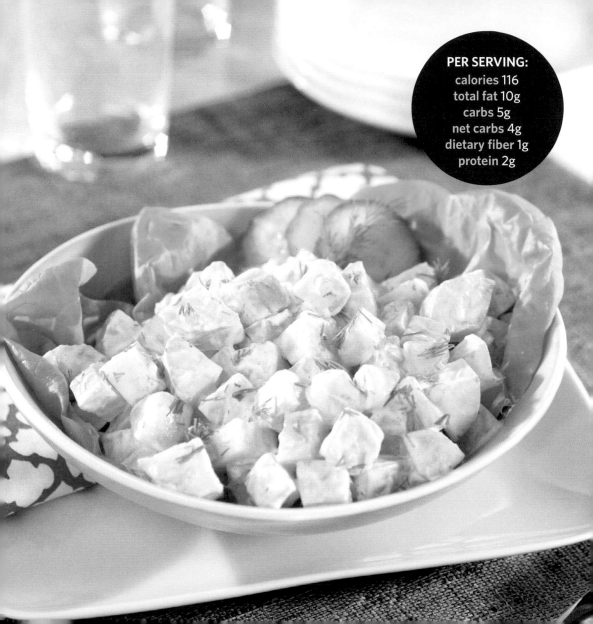

PER SERVING:
calories 116
total fat 10g
carbs 5g
net carbs 4g
dietary fiber 1g
protein 2g

Smoky Kale Chiffonade

MAKES 4 SERVINGS

12 ounces fresh young kale or
     mustard greens
 3 slices bacon

 2 tablespoons crumbled blue
     cheese

1. Rinse kale well in large bowl of warm water; drain in colander. Discard any discolored leaves; trim away tough stem ends. To prepare chiffonade, stack leaves and tightly roll up. Slice crosswise into ½-inch slices; separate into strips. Set aside.

2. Cook bacon in medium skillet over medium heat until crisp. Remove bacon to paper towel. Remove all but 1 tablespoon drippings.

3. Add kale to drippings in skillet. Cook and stir over medium-high heat 2 to 3 minutes until wilted and tender (older leaves may take slightly longer).

4. Crumble bacon. Toss bacon and blue cheese with kale. Transfer to warm serving dish. Serve immediately.

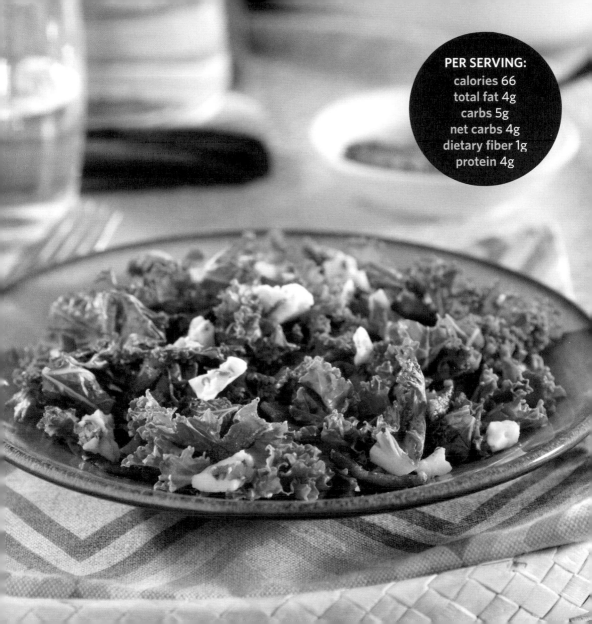

Broccoli Italian Style

MAKES 4 SERVINGS

1¼ **pounds fresh broccoli**
2 **tablespoons lemon juice**
1 **teaspoon extra virgin olive oil**
1 **clove garlic, minced**

1 **teaspoon chopped fresh Italian parsley**
Dash black pepper

1. Trim broccoli, discarding tough stems. Cut broccoli into florets with 2-inch stems. Peel remaining stems; cut into ½-inch slices.

2. Bring 1 quart water to a boil in large saucepan over medium-high heat. Add broccoli; return to a boil. Cook 3 to 5 minutes or until broccoli is tender. Drain; transfer to serving dish.

3. Combine lemon juice, oil, garlic, parsley and pepper in small bowl. Pour over broccoli; toss to coat. Cover and let stand 1 hour before serving to allow flavors to blend. Serve at room temperature.

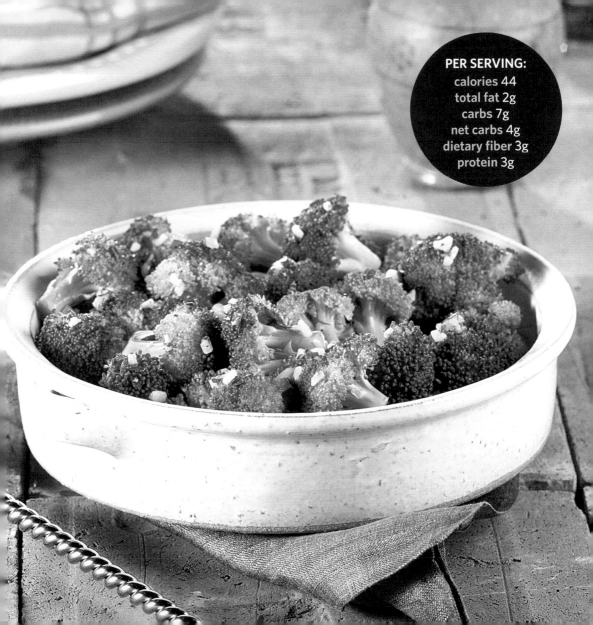

PER SERVING:
calories 44
total fat 2g
carbs 7g
net carbs 4g
dietary fiber 3g
protein 3g

Dilled Brussels Sprouts

MAKES 3 SERVINGS

1 package (10 ounces) frozen brussels sprouts *or* 1 pint fresh brussels sprouts

½ cup beef broth

1 teaspoon dill seed

1 teaspoon dried minced onion

Salt and black pepper

1. Combine brussels sprouts, broth, dill and onion in medium saucepan. Bring to a simmer over medium heat. Reduce heat to medium-low; cover and simmer 8 to 10 minutes or until sprouts are nearly tender.

2. Uncover and continue to simmer until most of liquid is evaporated. Season with salt and pepper.

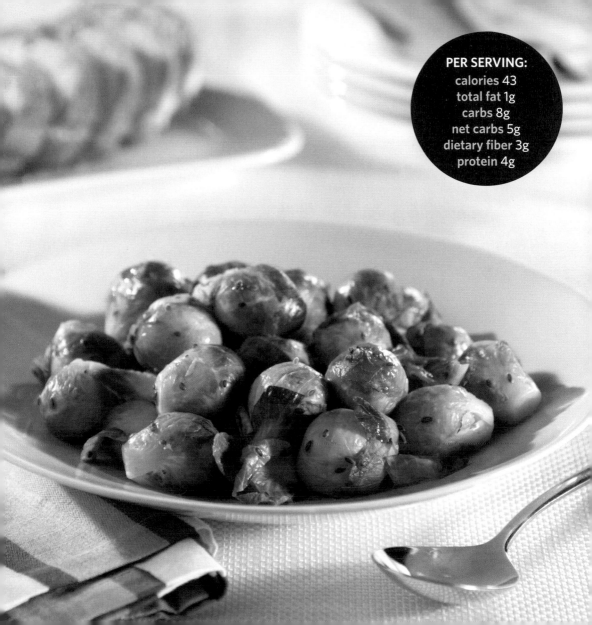

PER SERVING:
calories 43
total fat 1g
carbs 8g
net carbs 5g
dietary fiber 3g
protein 4g

Crab Spinach Salad
with Tarragon Dressing

MAKES 4 SERVINGS

12 ounces coarsely flaked cooked crabmeat *or* 2 packages (6 ounces each) frozen crabmeat, thawed and drained

1 cup chopped tomatoes

1 cup sliced cucumber

⅓ cup sliced red onion

¼ cup mayonnaise

¼ cup sour cream

¼ cup chopped fresh parsley

2 tablespoons milk

2 teaspoons chopped fresh tarragon *or* ½ teaspoon dried tarragon leaves

1 clove garlic, minced

¼ teaspoon hot pepper sauce

8 cups fresh spinach

1. Combine crabmeat, tomatoes, cucumber and onion in medium bowl. Combine mayonnaise, sour cream, parsley, milk, tarragon, garlic and hot pepper sauce in small bowl.

2. Line four salad plates with spinach. Place crabmeat mixture on spinach; drizzle with dressing.

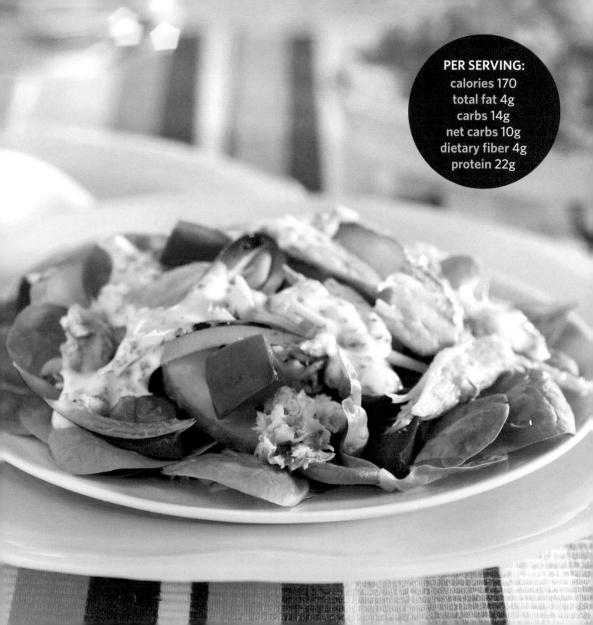

PER SERVING:
calories 170
total fat 4g
carbs 14g
net carbs 10g
dietary fiber 4g
protein 22g

Creamed Kale

MAKES 8 SERVINGS

2 large bunches kale (about 2 pounds)

2 tablespoons butter

2 tablespoons almond flour

1½ cups milk

½ cup shredded Parmesan cheese, plus additional for garnish

2 cloves garlic, minced

¼ teaspoon salt

⅛ teaspoon ground nutmeg

1. Remove stems from kale; discard. Coarsely chop leaves. Bring large saucepan of water to a boil. Add kale; cook 5 minutes. Drain.

2. Melt butter in large saucepan over medium heat. Whisk in almond flour; cook 1 minute, stirring constantly. Gradually whisk in milk until well blended. Cook 4 to 5 minutes or until sauce boils and thickens, whisking constantly. Whisk in ½ cup cheese, garlic, salt and nutmeg. Remove from heat. Stir in kale. Sprinkle with additional cheese, if desired.

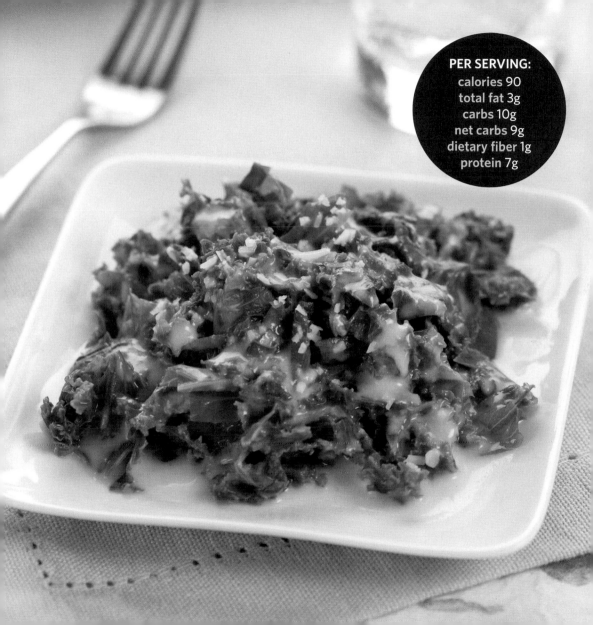

Red Cabbage with Bacon and Mushrooms

MAKES 6 SERVINGS

5 slices thick-cut bacon, chopped (about 8 ounces)

1 onion, chopped

1 package (8 ounces) cremini mushrooms, chopped (½-inch pieces)

¾ teaspoon dried thyme

½ medium red cabbage, cut into wedges, cored and then cut crosswise into ¼-inch slices (about 7 cups)

¾ teaspoon salt

¼ teaspoon black pepper

⅔ cup chicken broth

3 tablespoons cider vinegar

¼ cup chopped walnuts, toasted*

3 tablespoons chopped fresh parsley

To toast walnuts, cook in small skillet over medium heat 4 to 5 minutes or until lightly browned, stirring frequently.

1. Cook bacon in large saucepan or skillet over medium-high heat until crisp. Drain on paper towels.

2. Add onion to saucepan; cook and stir 5 minutes or until softened. Add mushrooms and thyme; cook about 6 minutes or until mushrooms begin to brown, stirring occasionally. Add cabbage, ¾ teaspoon salt and ¼ teaspoon pepper; cook about 7 minutes or until cabbage has wilted.

3. Stir in broth, vinegar and half of bacon; bring to a boil. Reduce heat to low; cook, uncovered, 15 to 20 minutes or until cabbage is tender.

4. Stir in walnuts and parsley; season with additional salt and pepper if necessary. Sprinkle with remaining bacon.

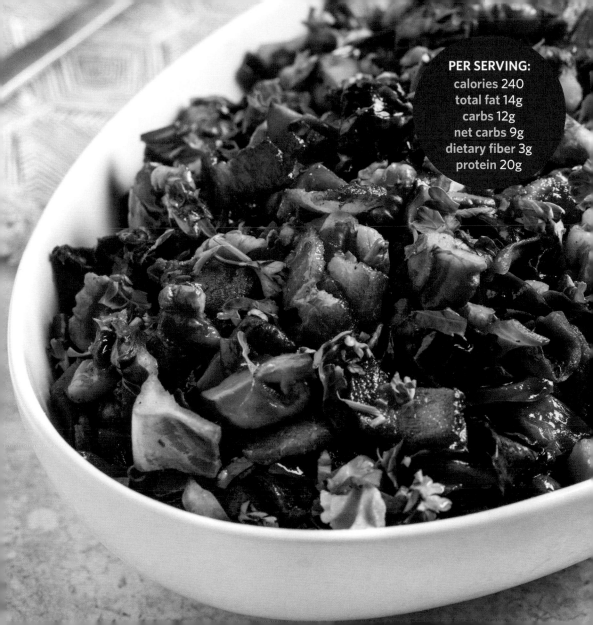

PER SERVING:
calories 240
total fat 14g
carbs 12g
net carbs 9g
dietary fiber 3g
protein 20g

Green Goddess Cobb Salad

MAKES 6 SERVINGS

PICKLED ONIONS
- 1 cup thinly sliced red onion
- ½ cup white wine vinegar
- ¼ cup water
- 1 teaspoon salt

DRESSING
- 1 cup mayonnaise
- 1 cup fresh Italian parsley leaves
- 1 cup baby arugula
- ¼ cup extra virgin olive oil
- 3 tablespoons lemon juice
- 3 tablespoons minced fresh chives
- 2 tablespoons fresh tarragon leaves

- 1 clove garlic, minced
- 1 teaspoon Dijon mustard
- ½ teaspoon salt
- ⅛ teaspoon black pepper

SALAD
- 4 eggs
- 4 cups Italian salad blend (romaine and radicchio)
- 2 cups chopped stemmed kale
- 2 cups baby arugula
- 2 avocados, sliced and halved
- 2 tomatoes, cut into wedges
- 2 cups cooked chicken strips
- 1 cup chopped crisp-cooked bacon

1. For pickled onions, combine onion, vinegar, ¼ cup water and 1 teaspoon salt in large glass jar. Seal jar; shake well. Refrigerate at least 1 hour or up to 1 week.

2. For dressing, combine mayonnaise, parsley, 1 cup arugula, oil, lemon juice, chives, tarragon, garlic, mustard, ½ teaspoon salt and pepper in blender or food processor; blend until smooth, stopping to scrape down side once or twice. Transfer to jar; refrigerate until ready to use. Just before serving, thin dressing with 1 to 2 tablespoons water, if necessary, to reach desired consistency.

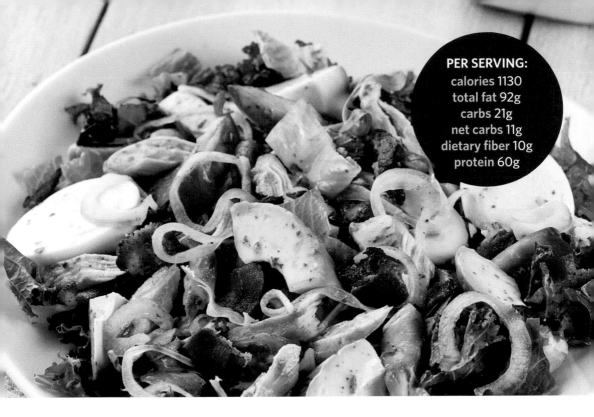

PER SERVING:
calories 1130
total fat 92g
carbs 21g
net carbs 11g
dietary fiber 10g
protein 60g

3. Fill medium saucepan with water; bring to a boil over high heat. Carefully lower eggs into water. Reduce heat to medium; boil gently 12 minutes. Drain eggs; add cold water and ice cubes to saucepan to cool eggs. When eggs are cool enough to handle, peel and cut into halves or quarters.

4. For salad, combine salad blend, kale, 2 cups arugula and pickled onions in large bowl; divide among 6 serving bowls. Top each salad with avocados, tomatoes, chicken, bacon and eggs. Top with ¼ cup dressing; toss to coat.

Brussels Sprouts with Bacon and Butter

MAKES 4 SERVINGS

6 slices thick-cut bacon, cut into ½-inch pieces

1½ pounds brussels sprouts (about 24 medium), halved

¼ teaspoon salt

¼ teaspoon black pepper

2 tablespoons butter, softened

1. Preheat oven to 375°F. Cook bacon in medium skillet until almost crisp. Drain on paper towels; set aside. Reserve 1 tablespoon drippings for cooking brussels sprouts.

2. Place brussels sprouts on large baking sheet. Drizzle with reserved bacon drippings and sprinkle with ¼ teaspoon salt and ¼ teaspoon pepper; toss to coat. Spread in single layer on baking sheet.

3. Roast 30 minutes or until brussels sprouts are browned and crispy, stirring once.

4. Place brussels sprouts in large bowl; stir in butter until completely coated. Stir in bacon; season with additional salt and pepper.

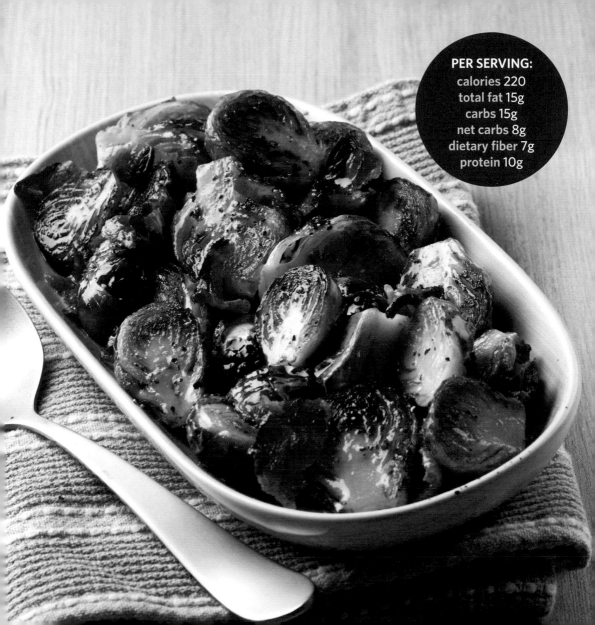

PER SERVING:
calories 220
total fat 15g
carbs 15g
net carbs 8g
dietary fiber 7g
protein 10g

Steakhouse Chopped Salad

MAKES 10 SERVINGS (20 CUPS)

DRESSING
- 1 package (about 2 tablespoons) Italian salad dressing mix
- ⅓ cup white balsamic vinegar
- ¼ cup Dijon mustard
- ⅔ cup extra virgin olive oil

SALAD
- 1 medium head iceberg lettuce, chopped
- 1 medium head romaine lettuce, chopped
- 1 can (about 14 ounces) artichoke hearts, quartered lengthwise then sliced crosswise
- 1 large avocado, diced
- 1½ cups crumbled blue cheese
- 2 hard-cooked eggs, chopped
- 1 ripe tomato, chopped
- ½ small red onion, finely chopped
- 12 slices bacon, crisp-cooked and crumbled

1. For dressing, whisk salad dressing mix, vinegar and mustard in medium bowl. Slowly whisk in oil in thin steady stream. Set aside until ready to use. (Dressing can be made up to 1 week in advance; refrigerate in jar with tight-fitting lid.)

2. For salad, combine lettuces, artichokes, avocado, cheese, eggs, tomato, onion and bacon in large bowl. Add dressing; toss to coat.

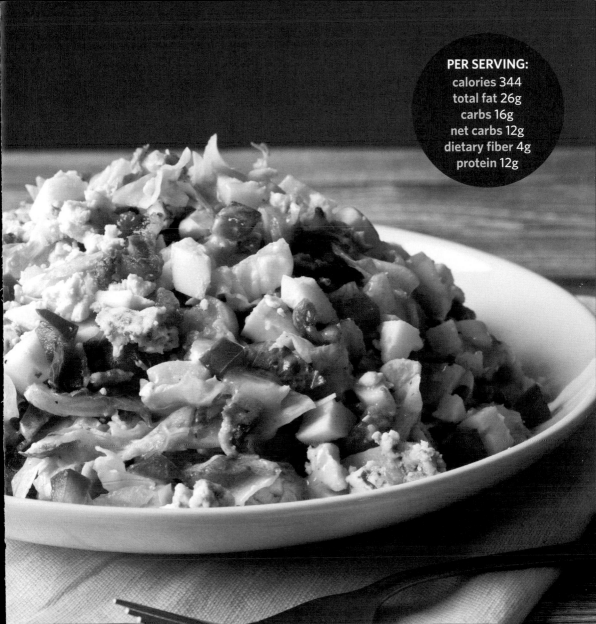

Zoodles in Tomato Sauce

MAKES 8 SERVINGS

3 teaspoons olive oil, divided

2 cloves garlic

1 tablespoon tomato paste

1 can (28 ounces) whole tomatoes, undrained

1 teaspoon dried oregano

½ teaspoon salt

2 large zucchini (about 16 ounces each), ends trimmed, cut into 3-inch pieces

¼ cup shredded Parmesan cheese

1. Heat 2 teaspoons oil in medium saucepan over medium heat. Add garlic; cook 1 minute or until fragrant but not browned. Stir in tomato paste; cook 30 seconds, stirring constantly. Add tomatoes with juice, oregano and salt; break up tomatoes with wooden spoon. Bring to a simmer. Reduce heat; cook 30 minutes or until thickened.

2. Meanwhile, spiral zucchini with fine spiral blade of spiralizer. Heat remaining 1 teaspoon oil in large skillet over medium-high heat. Add zucchini; cook 4 to 5 minutes or until tender, stirring frequently. Transfer to serving plates; top with tomato sauce and Parmesan, if desired.

NOTE: If you don't have a spiralizer, cut the zucchini into ribbons with a mandoline or sharp knife. Or purchase 2 pounds of precut zucchini noodles from the produce section of the supermarket.

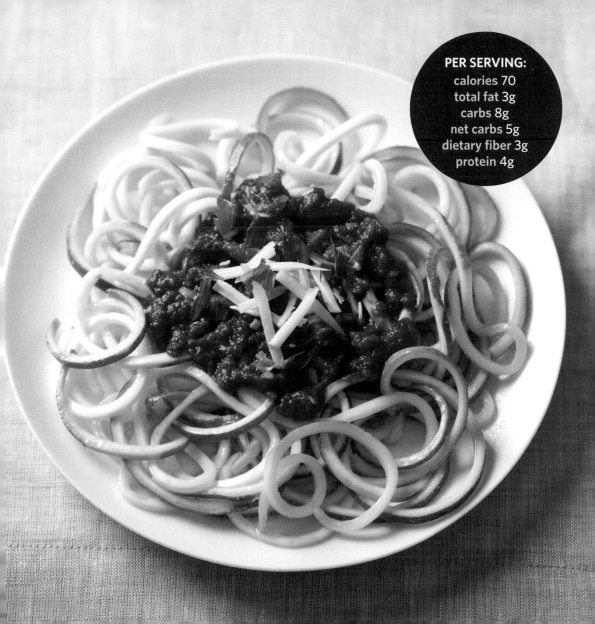

PER SERVING:
calories 70
total fat 3g
carbs 8g
net carbs 5g
dietary fiber 3g
protein 4g

Wedge Salad

MAKES 4 SERVINGS

DRESSING

- ¾ cup mayonnaise
- ½ cup buttermilk
- 1 cup crumbled blue cheese, divided
- 1 clove garlic, minced
- ⅛ teaspoon onion powder
- ⅛ teaspoon salt
- ⅛ teaspoon ground black pepper

SALAD

- 1 head iceberg lettuce
- 1 large tomato, diced (about 1 cup)
- ½ small red onion, cut into thin rings
- ½ cup crumbled crisp-cooked bacon (6 slices)

1. For dressing, combine mayonnaise, buttermilk, ½ cup cheese, garlic, onion powder, salt and pepper in food processor or blender; process until smooth.

2. For salad, cut lettuce into quarters through stem end; remove stem from each wedge. Place wedges on individual serving plates; top with dressing. Sprinkle with tomato, onion, remaining ½ cup cheese and bacon.

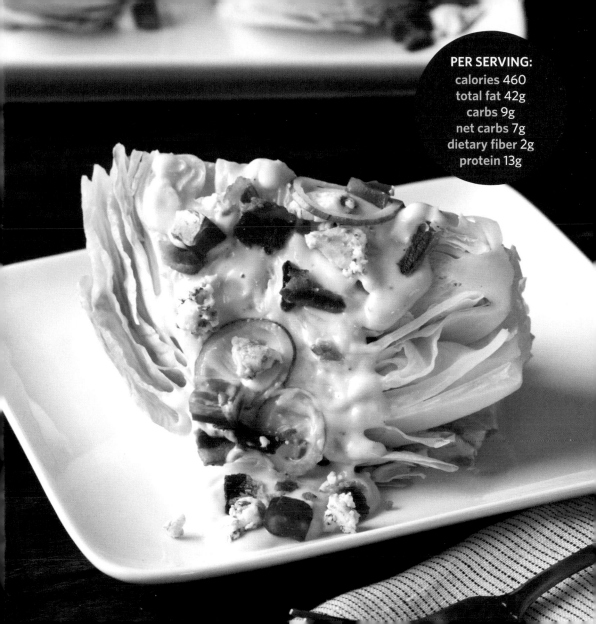

Mashed Cauliflower

2 heads cauliflower (to equal
   8 cups florets)
1 tablespoon butter

1 tablespoon half-and-half or
   whipping cream
Salt

1. Break cauliflower into equal-size florets. Place in large saucepan in about 2 inches of water. Simmer over medium heat 20 to 25 minutes, or until cauliflower is very tender and falling apart. (Check occasionally to make sure there is enough water to prevent burning; add water if necessary.) Drain well.

2. Place cooked cauliflower in food processor or blender. Process until almost smooth. Add butter. Process until smooth, adding half-and-half as needed to reach desired consistency. Season with salt to taste.

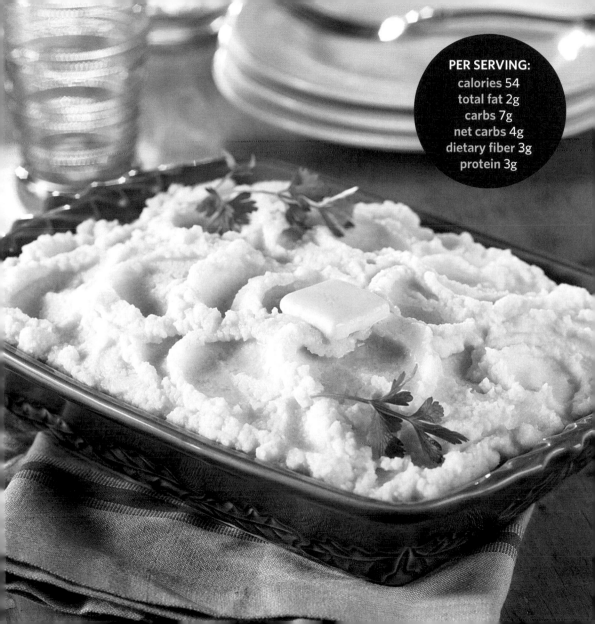

Zucchini with Feta Casserole

MAKES 4 SERVINGS

4 medium zucchini
1 tablespoon butter
2 eggs, beaten
½ cup grated Parmesan cheese
⅓ cup crumbled feta cheese
2 tablespoons chopped fresh parsley

2 teaspoons chopped fresh marjoram
Dash hot pepper sauce
Salt and black pepper

1. Preheat oven to 375°F. Spray 2-quart casserole with nonstick cooking spray.

2. Grate zucchini; drain in colander. Melt butter in large skillet over medium heat. Add zucchini; cook and stir until slightly browned.

3. Remove from heat; stir in eggs, cheeses, parsley, marjoram, hot pepper sauce, salt and black pepper until well blended. Pour into prepared casserole.

4. Bake 35 minutes or until hot and bubbly.

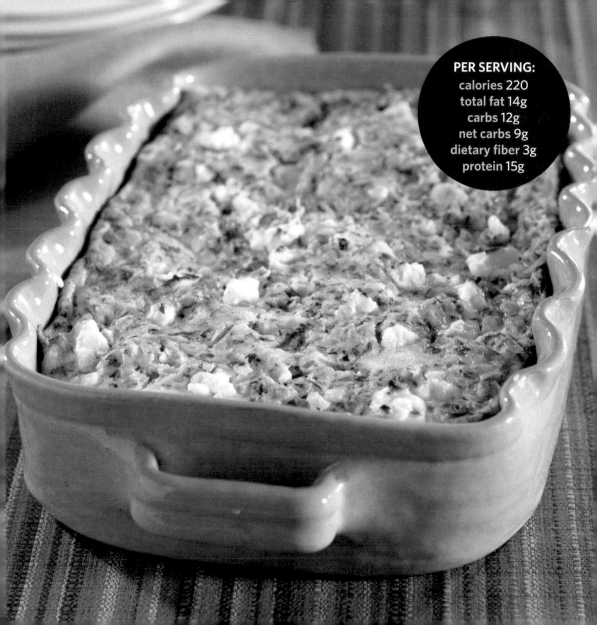

PER SERVING:
calories 220
total fat 14g
carbs 12g
net carbs 9g
dietary fiber 3g
protein 15g

Greek Salad

MAKES 6 SERVINGS

SALAD

3 medium tomatoes, cut into 8 wedges each and seeds removed

1 green bell pepper, cut into 1-inch pieces

½ English cucumber (8 to 10 inches), quartered lengthwise and sliced crosswise

½ red onion, thinly sliced

½ cup pitted kalamata olives

1 block (8 ounces) feta cheese, cut into ½-inch cubes

DRESSING

6 tablespoons extra virgin olive oil

3 tablespoons red wine vinegar

1 to 2 cloves garlic, minced

¾ teaspoon dried oregano

¾ teaspoon salt

¼ teaspoon black pepper

1. Combine tomatoes, bell pepper, cucumber, onion and olives in large bowl. Top with feta.

2. For dressing, whisk oil, vinegar, garlic, oregano, salt and pepper in medium bowl until well blended. Pour over salad; stir gently to coat.

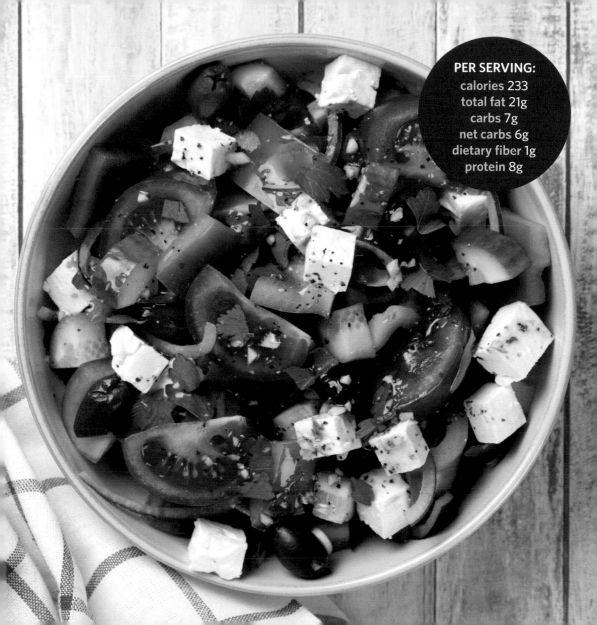

PER SERVING:
calories 233
total fat 21g
carbs 7g
net carbs 6g
dietary fiber 1g
protein 8g

Asparagus with Creamy Garlic Dressing

MAKES 4 SERVINGS

2 tablespoons sour cream
1 tablespoon buttermilk or whipping cream
1 teaspoon grated lemon peel
1 clove garlic, minced

Salt and black pepper
24 asparagus spears, trimmed and diagonally sliced into 1-inch pieces

1. Whisk sour cream, buttermilk, lemon peel and garlic in small bowl. Season with salt and pepper.

2. Place asparagus in large skillet; add enough water to just cover asparagus and season with salt. Bring to a boil over high heat. Reduce heat to a simmer; cook 3 to 5 minutes or until asparagus is crisp-tender. Drain and rinse under cold water to stop cooking. Place in serving bowl. Add dressing; stir until well coated.

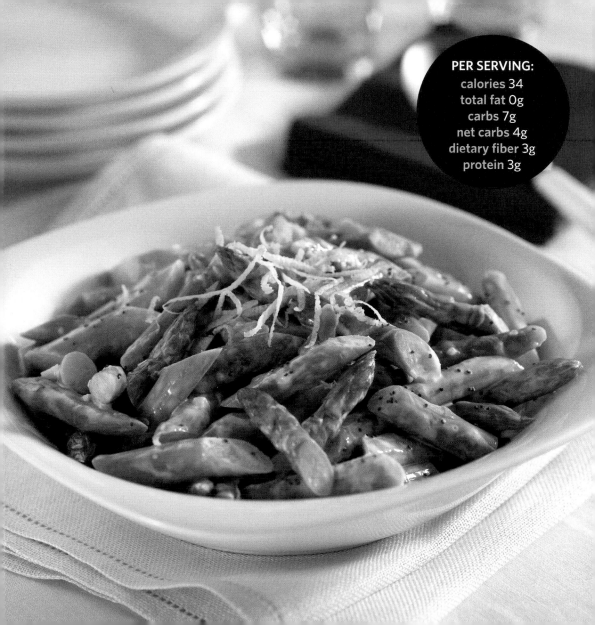

PER SERVING:
calories 34
total fat 0g
carbs 7g
net carbs 4g
dietary fiber 3g
protein 3g

Layered Caprese Salad

MAKES 4 SERVINGS

2 tablespoons extra virgin
   olive oil

2 teaspoons balsamic vinegar

2 cloves garlic, minced
   Salt and black pepper

½ small red onion, thinly sliced

3 medium tomatoes, sliced

½ cup (2 ounces) shredded
   mozzarella cheese

2 tablespoons chopped fresh
   parsley

2 tablespoons shredded fresh
   basil

1. Whisk oil, vinegar, garlic, salt and pepper in small bowl until well blended.

2. Spread half of onion in serving dish. Layer with half of tomatoes and sprinkle with half of cheese, parsley and basil. Drizzle with half of dressing. Repeat layers of onions, tomatoes, herbs and dressing. Serve at room temperature or cover and refrigerate 1 hour.

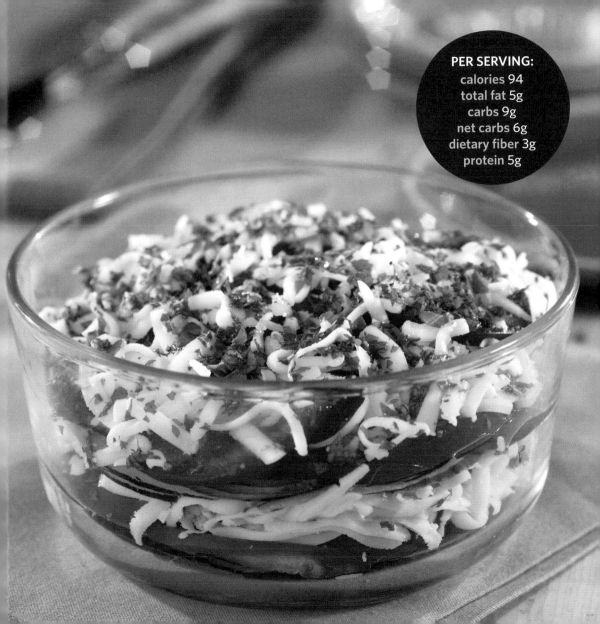

Metric Conversion Chart

VOLUME MEASUREMENTS (dry)

1/8 teaspoon = 0.5 mL
1/4 teaspoon = 1 mL
1/2 teaspoon = 2 mL
3/4 teaspoon = 4 mL
1 teaspoon = 5 mL
1 tablespoon = 15 mL
2 tablespoons = 30 mL
1/4 cup = 60 mL
1/3 cup = 75 mL
1/2 cup = 125 mL
2/3 cup = 150 mL
3/4 cup = 175 mL
1 cup = 250 mL
2 cups = 1 pint = 500 mL
3 cups = 750 mL
4 cups = 1 quart = 1 L

VOLUME MEASUREMENTS (fluid)

1 fluid ounce (2 tablespoons) = 30 mL
4 fluid ounces (1/2 cup) = 125 mL
8 fluid ounces (1 cup) = 250 mL
12 fluid ounces (1 1/2 cups) = 375 mL
16 fluid ounces (2 cups) = 500 mL

WEIGHTS (mass)

1/2 ounce = 15 g
1 ounce = 30 g
3 ounces = 90 g
4 ounces = 120 g
8 ounces = 225 g
10 ounces = 285 g
12 ounces = 360 g
16 ounces = 1 pound = 450 g

DIMENSIONS

1/16 inch = 2 mm
1/8 inch = 3 mm
1/4 inch = 6 mm
1/2 inch = 1.5 cm
3/4 inch = 2 cm
1 inch = 2.5 cm

OVEN TEMPERATURES

250°F = 120°C
275°F = 140°C
300°F = 150°C
325°F = 160°C
350°F = 180°C
375°F = 190°C
400°F = 200°C
425°F = 220°C
450°F = 230°C

BAKING PAN SIZES

Utensil	Size in Inches/Quarts	Metric Volume	Size in Centimeters
Baking or Cake Pan (square or rectangular)	8×8×2	2 L	20×20×5
	9×9×2	2.5 L	23×23×5
	12×8×2	3 L	30×20×5
	13×9×2	3.5 L	33×23×5
Loaf Pan	8×4×3	1.5 L	20×10×7
	9×5×3	2 L	23×13×7
Round Layer Cake Pan	8×1½	1.2 L	20×4
	9×1½	1.5 L	23×4
Pie Plate	8×1¼	750 mL	20×3
	9×1¼	1 L	23×3
Baking Dish or Casserole	1 quart	1 L	—
	1½ quart	1.5 L	—
	2 quart	2 L	—